Psychological and Medical Aspects of Induced Abortion

Recent Titles in
Bibliographies and Indexes in Women's Studies

Women in China: A Selected and Annotated Bibliography
Karen T. Wei

Women Writers of Spain: An Annotated Bio-Bibliographical Guide
Carolyn L. Galerstein and Kathleen McNerney, editors

The Equal Rights Amendment: An Annotated Bibliography of the Issues,
1976-1985
Renee Feinberg, compiler

Childbearing Among Hispanics in the United States: An
Annotated Bibliography
Katherine F. Darabi, compiler

Women Writers of Spanish America: An Annotated Bibliographical Guide
Diane E. Marting, editor

Women in Ireland: An Annotated Bibliography
Anna Brady, compiler

PSYCHOLOGICAL AND MEDICAL ASPECTS OF INDUCED ABORTION

A Selective, Annotated Bibliography, 1970-1986

Compiled by
Eugenia B. Winter

Bibliographies and Indexes in Women's Studies,
Number 7

GREENWOOD PRESS
NEW YORK • WESTPORT, CONNECTICUT • LONDON

Library of Congress Cataloging-in-Publication Data

Winter, Eugenia B.
   Psychological and medical aspects of induced abortion.

   (Bibliographies and indexes in women's studies,
ISSN 0742-6941 ; no. 7)
   Includes indexes.
   1. Abortion—Bibliography.   2. Abortion—Psychological
aspects—Bibliography.   I. Title.   II. Series.
Z6671.2.A2W56   1988   [RG734]   016.6188'8   88-194
ISBN 0-313-26100-8 (lib. bdg. : alk. paper)

British Library Cataloguing in Publication Data is available.

Library of Congress Catalog Card Number: 88-194
ISBN: 0-313-26100-8
ISSN: 0742-6941

First published in 1988

Greenwood Press, Inc.
88 Post Road West, Westport, Connecticut 06881

Printed in the United States of America

The paper used in this book complies with the
Permanent Paper Standard issued by the National
Information Standards Organization (Z39.48-1984).

10 9 8 7 6 5 4 3 2 1

For my sisters, Constance, Patricia, and Carole

Contents

Preface ix

Introduction xv

1. Abortion (General) 1

2. Abortion Clinics 16

3. Abortion Decision 32

4. Abortion Techniques (General) 48

5. Abortion Techniques (Specific) 55

6. Counseling 75

7. Morbidity and Mortality 84

8. Abortion Effects on Subsequent Pregnancy 92

9. Psychological Effects 101

10. Psychosocial Aspects 123

Author Index 129

Title Index 137

Subject Index 155

Preface

The researcher seeking material on the literature of the medical and psychological aspects of induced abortion published between 1970 and 1986 is faced with a multitude of books and articles scattered throughout a vast array of publications ranging from popular periodicals to medical textbooks. Although there have been bibliographic guides published previously, the citations have not been annotated or were annotated only very briefly. This guide aims to correct this problem in this area of extreme interest and importance.

Because the literature is so extensive, I have selected to annotate five hundred titles that are either classics in the field or representational of the kinds of writing being published on the subjects of interest. In addition, included within the five hundred title limitation are a number of audiovisual items. Here again, bibliographic data has been scanty or nonexistent. I have previewed all of the films, video, and audio recordings that are in the guide.

I have intentionally concentrated on research materials originally published in English, although there are a number of works translated into English from other languages. These works were deemed too significant in terms of their influence on the field to leave out. In particular, Japan, Sweden, and several eastern European countries have produced important research cited in this guide.

TIME PERIOD COVERED

This book covers material written or produced during the 1970-1986 period. In the United States, prior to the Roe vs. Wade decision of 1973, the abortion literature reflects the difficulties physicians and patients alike were having dealing with induced abortion. State laws (Colorado, 1967; California, 1967; Georgia, 1968; Hawaii, 1970; New York, 1970; and twelve others) did not entirely make abortion accessible. Change was slow, and access was often limited to the financially privileged (Smith, E. Dorsey, p. 5).

During this pre-Supreme Court decision period a number of articles were written discussing how women could "qualify" for abortions, usually by psychiatric evaluation by a panel of doctors. The other option was, of course, illegal abortion. Citations on morbidity and mortality statistics from this period will prove illuminating.

Literature from the 1970-1973 period also shows the efforts of physicians from all medical specialties to help change restrictive laws. In addition, draft statements by influential professional groups had an impact on the changing medical climate towards abortion and these are cited in this book.

TERMINOLOGY

The term "induced abortion," as used in defining which citations are included in this guide, covers elective (voluntary) abortion, or "the interruption of pregnancy before viability at the request of the woman but not for reasons of impaired maternal health or fetal disease" (Pritchard, p. 477). Thus material on induced abortion for genetic indications is not included. (Such literature is broadly based and would include such areas as testing, genetic screening, laboratory analysis techniques, the decision-making process, as well as many of the same medical techniques used for induced abortion for nongenetic indications).

In addition, it should be noted that a number of other terms have been used, accurately and sometimes inaccurately, by the medical and lay communities for "induced abortion," such as "therapeutic abortion," "legal abortion," "miscarriage," and so forth. I have consciously avoided using these terms, instead utilizing "induced abortion" whenever possible.

Terminology confusion also exists in the area of abortion techniques. For example, "vacuum aspiration" is sometimes also called "vacuum curettage," "suction curettage," "vacuum extraction," and "vacuum aspiration." In general, I have placed the citation in the detailed subject index under the term used by the author, with cross references when appropriate.

Abortion is an emotional as well as a medical and psychological issue, and the terminology surrounding abortion is equally charged with emotion-laden words. I have tried to avoid using vocabulary that favors certain viewpoints. Thus, antiabortion terms such as "mother" for "pregnant woman," "child" for "fetus" and "prolife" for antiabortion" have been omitted, as have proabortion words such as "prochoice" or "products of conception" for "fetus."   These distinctions may appear irrelevant for some.

Authorial bias is equally possible with abortion material. In general, the majority of the citations are written by scientists or physicians who present the facts with no indication of authorial bias.   In several cases I have included examples of proabortion or antiabortion literature because of its importance or notoriety. In such cases bias will be indicated. I have also avoided making evaluative comments about each citation except where the work is especially outstanding or problematic. Although it was not possible to exclude technical or medical vocabulary, I have tried to annotate clearly enough to   make the citations accessible to a wide audience.

ARRANGEMENT AND INDEXES

The book is divided into ten broad subject areas to permit easy access to the material.   For example, a researcher interested in counseling of abortion patients can quickly scan the "counseling" section.   If specific material on counseling techniques such as group therapy is needed, the detailed subject index at the back will lead directly to the available citation(s).   The author, title, and subject indexes all access material by citation number rather than by page

Some citations may appear to be placed in rather peripheral sections, but this is deliberate in order to avoid having more than ten major subject divisions.   I have thus used frequent "see" and "see also" references to alert readers to the fact that material may appear in related subject categories.

REVIEW OF THE LITERATURE

It is not my intention to reiterate current trends in abortion research. However, I do want to highlight for the researcher the most important literature reviews included in the guide that will serve as excellent starting points for further study.

If I had to choose one title that is the most valuable tool for general abortion research, it would be Christopher Tietze's Induced Abortion: A World Review (65).   This statistical overview, edited by one of the preeminent experts in the field, covers nearly every aspect of induced abortion on an international scale from the public health, demographic and public policy points of view.

Friedlander et al's "Abortion: predicting the complexity of the decision-making process" (155) reviews and evaluates literature on the abortion decision.   Cornelia Friedman et al's early article "The decision-making process and the outcome of therapeutic abortion" (419) relates currrent literature to clinical experience.

There are a number of authors who have reviewed and evaluated literature on the psychological effects of abortion.   Jocelyn Handy (487) and Henry P. David (409) have both written helpful articles.   While the Hardy essay is more concerned with the British approach to the subject, David uses material from several countries to give a broader perspective.

Earlier review articles that should also prove useful are Robert Pasnau's "Psychiatric complications of therapeutic abortion" (451), Robert Jacques' "Abortion and psychological trauma" (425), G.S. Walter's "Psychologic and emotional consequences of elective abortion" (474), and Joy and Howard Osofsky's "Psychological reaction of patients to legalized abortion" (449).   Diana Brasher's "Abortion counseling" (303) evaluates counseling literature and indicates major issues in the field, while Leo Croghan reviews literature on potential psychological vulnerability connected with the new era of liberalized abortion (407).

Articles that   deal with a review of the literature of the psychosocial aspects of abortion are Karen Lodl et al's "Women's responses to abortion" (321), Lucy Olson's "Social and psychological correlates of pregnancy resolution among adolescent women" (496),   Illsley   and   Hall's "Psychosocial aspects of abortion: a review of issues and needed research "(491), and Lisa Shusterman's 1976 review, "The psychosocial factors of the abortion experience: a critical review" (498).

Michael Bracken deals with literature on the influence of a prior induced abortion on subsequent perinatal complications in his article (364), while C.J.R. Hogue systematically reviews the literature in "The effects of induced abortion on subsequent reproduction" (373).   Janet Daling's Ph.D. dissertation first reviews literature on subsequent pregnancy outcome, followed by data analysis (370).   Lynn Shalaby's 1975 Ph.D. dissertation, How Women Feel about Abortion: Psychological, Attitudinal and Physical Effects of Legal Abortion contains a literature review divided by three periods: pre-1966, before legal abortion;   from 1966-1972, when liberalization was beginning;   and after the Roe vs. Wade decision of February 22, 1973(464).

Two important, less frequently studied areas have received recent literature reviews.   Gibb and Millard's "Research on repeated abortion: state of the field 1973-1979" is a literature review followed by a study of methodological and data collection problems in current demographic studies (157).   Mark Randall Smith analyzes the relatively scanty number of studies of men and abortion in his 1979 Ph.D. dissertation, How Men who Accompany Women to the Abortion Service Perceive the Impact of Abortion upon Their Relationship and Themselves (468).

There are a number of articles dealing with a review of the literature of abortion techniques.   Margolis and Goldsmith's review of first-trimester literature (208) and Brenner's review of second-trimester literature (197) both appear in Progress in Gynecology, v. 6.   Susan Chaudry's "Pregnancy termination in midtrimester--review of major methods" (200) covers both methods and literature, while Edstrom's article evaluates literature and methods of the four midtrimester abortion methods (345). His 1979 article updates the 1975 one (346).   Nathanson reviews literature on abortifacient drugs(277).   King et al's "Abortion: practice and promise" (207) documents literature written during the 1970-1975 period.

ACKNOWLEDGMENTS

At California State College, Bakersfield, Lorna Frost and Dr.   Reza Azarmsa were extremely helpful in obtaining often elusive materials; Matt Hightower in dealing with the computer program and manuscript preparation;   and Rodney M. Hersberger in providing support for research activities.

Planned Parenthood Centers in Bakersfield and Los Angeles, the National Abortion Federation, Catholics for a Free Choice,   and Birthright of Bakersfield all provided research materials and helpful suggestions.

Thanks should also go to Dr. Howard L. Lachtman, Dr. Benton F. Scheide, and Dr. Thomas M. Watts for   advice and encouragement; Dr. Irwin C. Winter, for reviewing medical citations for accuracy;   Edward J. Lockman, for suggesting the importance of including material on the father; and Matthew E. Winter for his support throughout this project.

Introduction

The ten major subject divisions in the bibliography are:

Abortion (general)
Includes texts that cover current research on induced abortion from various perspectives. Types of works in this category are general in nature, covering aspects such as the legal or moral, in addition to the medical and psychological areas and often contain statistical overviews.

Abortion clinics
Focuses on setting up and maintaining standards for quality abortion clinics. Includes administrative and counseling aspects of clinics as well as medical concerns, attitudes and training for physicians and nurses in their work with abortion patients. Also covers access to abortions and availability of various kinds of hospitals, ambulatory, or free-standing clinics.

Abortion decision
Contains material on how women make the abortion decision, and how and why decisions are often delayed. Also contains material on repeat abortions.

Abortion techniques (general)
Concentrates on works that contain a number of techniques used in abortion, or works that compare and contrast various techniques, with accompanying medical complication rate data.

Abortion techniques (specific)
Material in this category will be more narrowly focused than in the section "Abortion techniques (general)." Examples of each kind of current abortion technique are included, with details on methods and results.

Counseling
Includes group therapy, counseling for partners and families, psychiatric evaluation, and social work. [See also **Psychological effects**].

Morbidity and Mortality
Focuses on statistical data on numbers of maternal deaths due to abortions. Also deals with comparisons of techniques in terms of their complication rates and relative risks.

Pregnancy, Abortion Effects on Subsequent
Contains material on the effects of induced abortion on subsequent reproductive outcomes.

Psychological effects
Material on pre-and postabortion psychological adjustments for both patient and families. Also covers contraceptive choice, patterns and use of birth control before and after abortion. [See also **Counseling**].

Psychosocial aspects
Includes epidemiological data on what kinds of women choose to have abortions and their socioeconomic backgrounds. Also includes psychosocial data on families or partners of patients.

Psychological and Medical Aspects of Induced Abortion

1

Abortion (General)

1. Amy, J.J. et al. "A suggested set of working definitions and criteria applicable to interruption of pregnancy." <u>Contraception.</u> 14.(1976): 193-197; bibl.
An international group of physicians suggests a uniform set of terms be adopted to use in studies of interruption of pregnancy in order to standardize data. Definitions include induction-abortion interval, successful abortion, cumulative abortion rates, complete and incomplete abortion.

2. Arnstein, Helene S. <u>What Every Woman Needs to Know About Abortion.</u> New York: Charles Scribner's Sons, 1973. 144 p.
A simple and clear account of the abortion decision process, techniques, psychological reactions and post-abortion contraception. Also contains list of sources for further information and a section on abortion alternatives.

3. Bluford, Robert Jr., and Petres, Robert E. <u>The Unwanted Pregnancy.</u> New York: Harper & Row, 1973. 116 p.
Using case studies, two men who counsel women on unwanted pregnancy discuss the background of a pregnancy decision. Contains sections on medical and moral aspects of abortion. Also discusses sources for obtaining abortions.

4. Bolognese, Roland J. et al. <u>Interruption of Pregnancy--A Total Patient</u>

Approach. Baltimore: Williams & Wilkins Company, 1975. 213 p.; bibl.
Provides chapters on demographic considerations, abortion techniques,
psychology of abortion, abortion counseling, indications for abortion,
management of fetal demise and concomitant sterilization.

5. The Boston Women's Health Book Collective.   The New Our Bodies,
Ourselves.   New York: Simon and Schuster, rev. ed., 1984.
Chapter 16 on the physical and emotional aspects of abortion covers
medical techniques, risks and complications, abortion facilities and
what happens   physically and emotionally during the procedures.
First-hand statements are given on various aspects of abortion
experiences.   Contains resource list of organizations and readings.

6. Bracken, Michael B. et al.   "Hospitalization for medical-legal and other
abortions in the U.S. 1970-1977."   American Journal of Public Health.
72.1 (January 1982): 30-37; bibl.
Study of national impact of the 1973 Supreme Court ruling on hospital
rates for all types of abortion and related rate of illegal abortion.   There
was a significant reduction in length of stay for spontaneous and other
abortion between 1970 and 1977.   This suggests decreasingly severe
symptomatology for complicated abortion.   The study also found that
during 1970-1977, illegal abortions were replaced by legal procedures.

7. Braude, Marjorie.   "The consequences of abortion legislation."   Women
and Therapy. 2.2-3 (Summer-Fall 1983): 81-90;   bibl.
Summarizes gains which women have made in terms of abortions and the
subsequent effects on both maternal and child health.   Also describes
changes in abortion climate due to those opposed to abortion.   Stresses
better education and improved contraceptive methods will help decrease
abortions rather than coercion.

8. Butler, J. Douglas, and Walbert, David F., eds.   Abortion. Medicine and
the Law. 3rd rev ed.   New York: Facts on File, 1986.   795 p.; bibl
Part Two, "Medicine," contains articles by leaders in the field on the
medical viewpoint on abortion practices, the effects on maternal health,
demographic an public health experience with legal abortion, the psychi-

atric implications and the impact of an abnormal fetus on the decision process. Appendices contain the 1973 Supreme Court decision.

9. Callahan, Daniel. Abortion: Law, Choice and Morality. New York: Macmillan,1970. 524 p.; bibl.
A thorough and scholarly analysis of all major issues related to abortion, using a theoretical and practical approach. Section I covers medical indications and medical sequelae, psychiatric indications and consequences and fetal indications for abortion.

10. Cates, Willard Jr. "Abortion as a treatment for unwanted pregnancy: the number two sexually-transmitted condition." Advances in Planned Parenthood. 12.(1978): 115-1211; bibl.
If unwanted pregnancy is classed as a venereal disease, it rates after gonorrhea as the most prevelant sexually-transmitted disease. First-trimester suction curettage is the preferred approach to legal abortion.   Presents statistics on incidence of unwanted pregnancy, treatment and safety and health comparisons.

11. Cates, Willard Jr.   "Legal abortion: the public health record." Science. 215.(March 26, 1982): 1586-90; bibl.
The availability of legal abortion in the U.S. has reduced deaths and surgical complications among women of childbearing age. It has also made possible the development of safer surgical procedures for pregnancy termination and increase the provision of low-cost outpatient gynecologic services.   There is some concern about potential adverse outcomes in later pregnancies and possibly higher risks of breast cancer in some women.

12. Chilman, Catherine S. Adolescent Sexuality in a Changing American Society: Social and Psychological Perspectives. DHEW Publication No. (NIH) 79-1426 . Bethesda, Md.: National Institutes of Health, 1979. pp. 184-188; bibl.
Chapter 8, "Abortion among adolescents," covers statistics for this age group, abortion risks, and a review of the major studies of characteristics of women who choose abortions. Also reviews literature

on psychological effects of abortion.

13. CIBA Foundation Symposium. <u>Abortion: Medical Progress and Social</u> <u>Implication.</u>   CIBA Foundation Symposium #115 .   New York: Wiley, 1986. 286 p.
A wide-ranging series of essays by an international group of specialists. Includes essays on sequelae of induced abortion, safety and effectiveness of various abortion methods, live-born infants of 24-28 weeks' gestation, post-abortion psychiatric hospitalization, and the effects of abortion on marriage.

14. Corsaro, Maria, and Korzeniowsky, Carole. <u>A Woman's Guide to Safe</u> <u>Abortion.</u> New York: Holt, Rinehart & Winston, 1983. 100 p.
An extremely clear guide to abortion. Covers descriptions of pregnancy tests how to choose an abortion facility, costs, insurance, abortion procedures, post-abortion precautions to avoid infections and contraception.   Includes appendices "If you're still not sure about abortion," Getting help," and a glossary.

15. Culliton, Barbara J. "Abortion: liberal laws do make abortion safe for women." <u>Science.</u> 188.(June 13, 1975): 1091.
Summary of a study carried out by the Institute of Medicine on legalized abortion and public health, which concludes that it is safer to have a legal abortion performed by a competent physician than it is to have an illegal abortion, and that it is safest to have a first trimester abortion. Under such circumstances there is little damage to the woman's health or psyche.

16. Denes, Magda. <u>In Necessity and Sorrow: Life and Death in an Abortion</u> <u>Hospital.</u> New York : Basic Books, 1976. 247 p.
Author records events which took place during her research at an abortion section of a New York hospital.   The resulting interviews with patients, physicians, clinic workers and friends or families of the patients show a wide range of coping techniques.

17. Denney, Myron K. <u>A Matter of Choice: An Essential Guide to Every</u>
<u>Aspect of Abortion.</u> New York: Simon and Schuster, 1983. 158 p.
A general guide to abortion, covering fetal development, alternatives,
roles of partners, doctors, counselors and emotional and medical aspects.
Also contains information on the "pro" and "anti" side of abortion and
contraceptive techniques.

18. Dornblaser, Carole, and Landy, Uta. <u>The Abortion Guide: A Handbook</u>
<u>for Women and Men.</u> New York: Playboy Press, 1982. 285 p.
General title which covers history of induced abortion, the abortion
decision,methods of abortion, psychological reactions, and contraception.
Includes personal accounts by women who have had abortions and a list
of clinics.

19. Ebon, Martin. <u>Every Woman's Guide to Abortion.</u>   New York: Universe
Books, 1971. 256 p.; bibl.
Contains information on where to get help, sources for guidance and case
histories.   Also contains texts of official statements by medical groups
on abortion.

20. Erlien, Marla et al. <u>More than a Choice: Women Talk About Abortion.</u>
Boston: Abortion Action Coalition, 1979. pam.;   24 p.
A general discussion about the abortion issue.   Contains personal
accounts of women who have had to consider the abortion option. Covers
economics, alternatives, sexuality and contraception.

21. Francome, Colin. <u>Abortion Practice in Britain and the U.S.</u>   London:
Allen & Unwin, 1986. 206 p.; bibl.
Begins with historical survey of abortion laws and practices in Britain
and the United States and compares the experience of legal abortion in
Britain since 1968 with the United States since 1970. Using official
data and questionnaires given to women in both countries, concludes that
a number of changes in social policy are indicated.   Improvements are
needed in sex education, birth control services, quality of relationship
between the sexes, and access to abortion services.

22. Gardner, Joy.   A Difficult Decision: A Compassionate Book about
Abortion.   Trumansburg, N.Y.: The Crossing Press, 1986. 115 p.; bibl.
Covers the abortion decision, alternatives to abortion, abortion and
politics,abortion procedures, aftercare and psychological effects and
coping techniques.

23. Gardner, R.F.R., and Stallworthy, J.A.   Abortion: The Personal
Dilemma.   Grand Rapids, Michigan: Wm. B. Eerdmans Pub. Co., 1972. 288 p.;
bibl.
Two British physicians examine the medical, social, and spiritual issues
about abortion.   Essays include ones on illegitimate pregnancy, the
pregnant student, mental and spiritual results of abortion, the decision,
and consequences when the abortion is refused.

24. Guttmacher, Alan F.   Pregnancy, Birth and Family Planning: A Guide
for Expectant Parents in the 1970's.   New York: The Viking Press, 1973.
365 p.
Chapter 10, "Miscarriage, Legal Abortion and Premature Labor," contains
a brief history of induced abortion, abortion techniques and research on
abortion.

25. Hafez, E.S.E., ed.   Voluntary Termination of Pregnancy.   Advances in
Reproductive Health Care Series .   England: MTP Press, Ltd., 1984. 178 p.
Essays by different contributors cover epidemiology, methodology of
various techniques, clinical aspects (including complications and effects
of abortion on subsequent pregnancies), and psychosocial aspects.

26. Hall, Robert E.   A Doctor's Guide to Having an Abortion.   New York:
New American Library, 1971. 68 p.
Reviews legal aspects of an abortion and how to go about finding a
physician.   Covers medical and psychological aspects and sterilization.

27. Hendin, David.   Everything you Need to Know about Abortion.   New
York: Pinnacle Books, 1971. 186 p.
Covers basic information about methods of contraception, the changing

abortion laws, ethical and religious considerations, and a question-and-answer section.

28. Henshaw, Stanley K. et al.   "Abortion services in the United States, 1979 and 1980." Family Planning Perspectives. 14.(1982): 5-15; bibl.
An analysis of data from the seventh national survey by The Alan Guttmacher Institute on all known providers of abortion services in the U.S. shows that in 1980 about one-quarter of all pregnancies were terminated by abortion.   Abortion services are still not readily available to all women, particularly those in nonmetropolitan areas. Three-fourths of all terminations took place in nonhospital facilities (nearly 80% as compared with fewer than 50% in 1973).

29. Hern, Warren. Abortion Practice.   Philadelphia: J.B. Lippincott Company, 1984. 340 p.; bibl.
A general textbook on abortion.   Covers epidemiology, patient screening and evaluation, counseling, operative procedures and techniques, staffing and operation techniques, long-term risks and program evaluation. Extensive   bibliographies.

30. Hern, Warren M., and Andrikopoulos, Bonnie, eds.   Abortion in the Seventies.   Western Regional Conference on Abortion, Proceedings. February 27-29, 1976.   New York: National Abortion Federation, 1977. 296 p.; bibl.
Transcripts from a major conference on abortion cover medical and public health aspects of abortion, evaluation of abortion services, abortion nursing, counseling and psychological aspects, economic and health insurance aspects, and legal, legislative and political aspects of abortion.   An important collection of essays from the foremost figures in the field.

31. Hilgers, Thomas W. et al.   New Perspectives on Human Abortion. Frederick, Md.: Aletheia Books, University Publications of America, Inc., 1981. 504 p.; bibl.
Contains 31 essays by doctors and laypersons on medical, legal, and social/philosophical issues on abortion from an anti-abortion point of

view.   Medical essays, among others, include: "Human Characteristics of
the Early Fetus: A Sonographic Demonstration;" "Medical and Ethical
Aspects of the Prenatal Diagnosis of Genetic Disease;" "Urologic
Complications of Legal Abortion," and "Sexual Assault and Pregnancy."

32. Hodgson, Jane E., ed. Abortion and Sterilization: Medical and Social
Aspects. London: Academic Press, 1981. 594 p.; bibl.
A definitive textbook on medical and social aspects of abortion and
sterilization.   Includes: epidemiology of induced abortion;   morbidity and
mortality statistics;   abortion and health;   abortion techniques;
prostaglandins;   sterilization techniques; vasectomy;   abortion services
in the U.S.; abortion and mental health.   Contains extensive
bibliographies.

33. Ide, Arthur F. Abortion Handbook: History, Clinical Practice and
Psychology of Abortion.   Las Colinas, Texas: Liberal Press, 1985. 152 p.
Contains essays on the medical and psychological aspects of abortion.
Also looks at the legal aspects and history of abortion in America.
Critiques "The   Silent Scream" from a pro-abortion point of view.

34. Institute of Medicine of the National Academy of Sciences. Legalized
Abortion and the Public Health. Washington, D.C., May 1975. 168 p.; bibl.
Committee reviews existing evidence on the relationship between
legalized abortion and the health of the public.   Covers medical and
demographic aspects of legal abortion in the U.S., abortion and the risk of
medical complications or death, psychological effects, birth defects and
selective abortion and contraception and abortion.   Appendices contain
summary of the Supreme Court decisions and a glossary of terms
associated with abortion.

35. It Happens to Us. Amalie R. Rothschild, producer/director. Film.   30
min. Karol Media, 1972.
An early (1972) film presents discussions with women of varying ages
who talk about their abortion experiences, both legal and illegal.
Includes brief explanation of medical techniques as well as statements
on safety and complication rates.

36. Keith, Louis G. et al., eds. The Safety of Fertility Reglulation. New York: Springer Publishing Company, 1980.   360 p.; bibl.
Chapter Five, "Pregnancy Termination," contains sections on menstrual regulation, prostaglandins, midtrimester abortion, abortion mortality, and reproduction after first-trimester induced abortion.

37. Kleinman, Ronald L. Induced Abortion. London: International Planned Parenthood Federation, 1972.   38 p.
A report of the IPPF Panel of Experts on Abortion covers definitions, incidence of induced abortion, socio-cultural aspects, abortion and family planning, techniques and side-effects and the relation between legislation and abortion practice.

38. Lane Committee.   Report of the Committee on the Working of the Abortion Act. London: HMSO, 1974. v.1, 288 p.; bibl. ; v.2, 271 p.; bibl.; v. 3, 109 p.; bibl.
A report studying the working of the Abortion Act in Great Britain discusses the case for and against abortion on demand and abortion on request and comes down in favor of the decision remaining a medical one. Makes a number of other recommendations, including both restrictive and liberalizing statutory amendment suggestions.

39. Legge, Jerome S. Abortion Policy: An Evaluation of the Consequences for Maternal Health.   Albany, New York: University of New York Press, 1985.   182 p.; bibl.
Analyzes abortion policy using advanced research designs and statistical techniques and case studies from the United States and Romania and Great Britain.   The most salient finding from the overall behavior of the health indicators is that health response to policy changes should not be conceptualized as a one-to-one relationship where conservative policy change results in health deterioration and vice versa.   Much depends upon the setting in which the change takes place, the timing of the policy intervention, the sexual culture of the society and its government's attitude toward contraception and other aspects of health.

40. Lewit, Sarah , ed. Abortion Techniques and Services: Proceedings of

the Conference. June 3-5, 1971. Amsterdam: Excerpta Medica, 1972.
211 p.; bibl.
Presents papers from a conference on abortion techniques and services.
Includes: medical aspects, legal aspects, social and administrative
aspects. Each set of papers is followed by a general discussion among
the participants. A useful review of 1971 thinking on all aspects of
abortion.

41. Moore-Cavar, Emily C. International Inventory of Information on
Induced Abortion. New York: Columbia University: Division of Social and
Administrative Sciences, International Institute for the Study of Human
Reproduction, 1973. 655 p.
An extremely useful summary of research on a wide range of topics,
including definitions, religion/ethical/moral aspects, medical and
psychological aspects, induced abortion and contraception, and
demographic aspects.

42. Morgentaler, Henry. Abortion and Contraception. Toronto : General
Publishing Company, 1982. 201 p.; bibl.
Covers basic facts about reproduction, including the dilemma of choice,
different methods of medical abortion, complications, psychological and
physical effects after an abortion, abortion and the law, and
contraception.

43. National Abortion Federation. Fact Sheet Series. Washington, D.C.,
1986-7. 6 p.
Bound series of informational sheets which answer common questions
and concerns about abortion. Titles in the series are: What is Abortion?;
Safety of Abortion; Who Have Abortions; Abortion after 12 Weeks;
Economics of Abortion; Public Support for Abortion.

44. Nazer, Isam R., editor. "Induced Abortion: A Hazard to Public
Health?" Proceedings of the First Conference of the IPPF Middle East and
North Africa Region. February, 1971. Beirut, Lebanon: International
Planned Parenthood Federation, 1971. 432 p.
An interesting group of papers from an international group of specialists

on various aspects of induced abortion.   Reports from different middle eastern countries explore socioeconomic trends.

45. Osofsky, Joy D. , and Osofsky, Howard J. The Abortion Experience: Psychological and Medical Impact. Hagerstown, Md.: Harper & Row, 1973. 668 p.; bibl.
A major compendium of detailed information on the medical, psychosocial, and legal aspects of abortion. Focuses on the U.S. experience but also contains international data where appropriate for the sake of comparison.   Also deals with future trends and needs for research. Essays are by a wide variety of physicians, social scientists and statisticians.

46. Petchesky, Rosalind P. Abortion and Woman's Choice: the State, Sexuality and Reproductive Freedom. Northeastern Series in Feminist Theory.   Boston: Northeastern University Press, 1984. 404 p.; bibl.
Study of women's reproductive rights from an ideological and sociological point of view.   Pertinent chapters are: "The social and economic conditions of women who get abortions;" "Considering the alternatives: the problems of contraception;" "Abortion and heterosexual culture: the teenage question;" and "Women's consciousness and the abortion decision."

47. Pipes, Mary. Understanding Abortion.   London: The Womans' Press Ltd., 1986. 181 p.; bibl.
Using personal accounts from 30 British women who underwent abortion, this book discusses the abortion decision, medical and psychological aspects, post-abortion adjustment and repeat abortions.   Contains list of resources in England.

48. Planned Parenthood of New York City, Inc.   Abortion: A Woman's Guide.   New York: Abeland Schuman, Ltd., 1973. Text by Beth R. Gutcheon; 147 p.
General, popularly written guide to the abortion decision, techniques, and contraception.

49. "Point Counterpoint." Washington, D.C.: Religious   Coalition for Abortion Rights, 1985.   26 p.; bibl.
Contains statistical data and information on contraceptive failure, abortion risks, psychological effects, fetal development, teenage pregnancy and amniocentesis.

50. Potts, Malcolm et al. <u>Abortion.</u>   Cambridge, England: Cambridge University Press, 1977. 575 p.; bibl.
A detailed survey of historical and medical aspects of abortion from a British viewpoint, but using comparative data from other countries. Chapter "Techniques of therapeutic abortion" gives history of various abortion techniques, morbidity statistics and psychological sequelae to abortion.

51. Pritchard, Jack A. et al. "Abortion." In   <u>Williams Obstetrics.</u>   17th ed. Norwalk, Ct.: Appleton-Century-Crofts, 1985.   pp. 467-490; bibl.
The classic medical textbook on obstetrics contains a concise outline and definitions for different kinds of abortions, including techniques used and management of complications.

52. Rudel, Harry W. et al. <u>Birth Control, Contraception, and Abortion.</u>
New York: The Macmillan Company, 1973. 372 p.; bibl.
A textbook designed for medical students and other health professionals. Methods of birth control are given greatest emphasis, such as hormonal contraception, intrauterine devices, and abortion.   Includes chapter on medical   and   psychiatric   indications   for   therapeutic   abortion, complications and medical sequelae, and medical techniques.   Cited references and suggested readings are given at the end of each chapter.

53. Saltman, Jules, and Zimering, Stanley.   <u>Abortion Today.</u> Springfield, Ill.: Charles C. Thomas, 1973. 175 p.; bibl.
Discusses definition of abortion, medical techniques, legal status, impact on women and families, costs and religious/moral arguments.

54. Schulder, Diane, and Kennedy, Florence. <u>Abortion Rap.</u> New York:

McGraw-Hill Book Company, 1971. 238 p.
Contains testimony from a number of women on their experiences with illegal abortions and what kinds of problems they encountered.

55. Sciarra, John J. et al., ed. Gynecology and Obstetrics. v. 6.   Rev ed.
Philadelphia: Harper and Row, 1986.
A looseleaf textbook which permits additions of new chapters where appropriate, this source is unusually comprehensive. Covers demography, maternal-child health, contraception, sterilization, diagnosis of pregnancy, abortion, psychosomatic problems and sexuality. Abortion chapter has sections ranging from general essays on induced abortion to long-term risks.

56. Sciarra, John J. et al., eds. Risks, Benefits and Controversies in Fertility Control.   Proceedings from Workshop on Risks, Benefits, and Controversies in Fertility Control.   March 13-16, 1977. Hagerstown, Md.: Harper & Row Pubs., 1978. 600 p.; bibl.
Section of volume dealing with pregnancy termination covers: menstrual regulation;   prostaglandin treatment; pharmacologic methods; cervical dilatation and other techniques for inducing abortion.   "Overview" identifies two major controversies: 1) safety of prostaglandin F2alpha as abortifacient and 2) the use of cervical dilatation and uterine evacuation as a method of abortion after the 12th week of pregnancy.

57. Scott, Michael J. Abortion: The Facts.   London: Darton, Longman and Todd, 1973. 62 p.
A review of the 1967 Abortion Act (Great Britain) from an anti-abortion point of view.   Discusses development of the fetus, medical and psychological effects, and socioeconomic factors.

58. Shapiro, Howard I. The Birth Control Book. New York: Avon Books, 1977. 356 p.; bibl.
Chapter 6, "Postcoital Contraception," and Chapter 7, "Abortion," give clear and concise descriptions of menstrual extraction and other abortion techniques such as saline and D & C abortions, and explains possible complications and psychological adjustment.

59. Siegel, Mark et al. <u>Abortion: An Eternal Social and Moral Issue.</u>
Plano, Texas: Information Aids, 1986. 88 p.
Reprinting documents from other sources, summarizes current
legislation and opinions on the abortion issue.   Contains a statistical
study of abortion in the U.S. and the rest of the world, with appendix
listing organizations which support abortion and those which oppose
abortion.

60. Skowronski, Marjory. <u>Abortion and Alternatives.</u>   Millbrae, Ca.: Les
Femmes Publishing, 1977. 145 p.; bibl.
Contains material on abortion and the law, differing perspectives on
abortion,medical and psychological consequences, the man's attitude
towards abortion, and contraception.   Suggested reading list follows the
text.

61. Sloane, R. Bruce, ed. <u>Abortion: Changing Views and Practice.</u>
Seminars in Psychiatry . New York: Grune & Stratton, 1971. 182 p.; bibl.
An excellent compendium of articles on a wide range of topics which
serves to show the state of the "transition period" immediately before
the 1973 Supreme Court decision.   Topics covered include attitudes
towards abortion, pro and con,psychological implications for therapeutic
abortion, socioeconomic aspects of abortion, and reviews of research and
studies.   An interesting, though controversial, article is Mildred Beck's
"Abortion: the mental health consequences of unwantedness."

62. Sloane, R. Bruce, and Horvitz, Diana F. <u>A General Guide to Abortion.</u>
Chicago: Nelson-Hall, 1973.
Covers legal history, abortion and the rights of women, socioeconomic
and international patterns of abortion seekers, and medical techniques.
Especially interesting is the Chapter,"Grounds for abortion: true and
false," which discusses various physical and medical indications for
abortion and which are accurate and which are not.

63. Smith, E. Dorsey. <u>Abortion: Health Care Perspectives.</u> Norwalk, Ct.:
Appleton-Century Crofts, 1972. 241 p.; bibl.
Written by a nurse at Mt. Sinai Medical Center, this general book exam-

ines social change and the historical evolution of abortion laws, physiology of pregnancy, methods of abortion, complications and follow-up care, contraception, attitudes and responses of women who seek abortions and their health care providers.

64. Tietze, Christopher. "Induced abortion, "In Handbook of Sexology. eds.   Money, John, and Musaph, Herman.   New York: Elsevier-North Holland, Inc., 1977. pp. 605-620; bibl.
Reports on incidence of abortion, legal status, procedures, complications, mortality, and effects of legislation on abortion.

65.   Tietze, Christopher. Induced Abortion: A World Review. 5th ed. A Population Council Fact Book. New York: The Population Council, 1983. 116 p.; bibl.
Presents overview of current international data on induced abortion, primarily from public health, demographic and public policy point of view.   Statistical tabulations make up the major part of the book, with the text providing background information.   Concise yet thorough analyses are given on medical statistics for repeat abortions, abortion procedures, period of gestation, complications, sequelae and mortality.

66. Zatuchni, Gerald I. et al., eds. Pregnancy Termination: Procedures, Safety and New Developments.   New York: Harper & Row, 1978. 447 p.; bibl.
Contains essays by 78 contributors who attended a workshop and postgraduate course on pregnancy termination.   Covers nearly every medical aspect of abortion, from early detection of pregnancy to late trimester pregnancy termination.   Also contains information on counseling and impact of illegal abortion.

2

Abortion Clinics

67. Abbott, Mildred I. et al. "The role of the nurse-midwife in an abortion evaluation clinic." Journal of Nurse Midwifery. 18.3 (Fall 1973): 17-22.
Describes a clinic where nurse-midwives participate in all aspects of abortion care, including antepartum, intrapartum, postpartum and family planning. Feels midwives are filling need for complete, supportive care of abortion patients.

68. Abortion Clinic. Frontline series. WGBH Educational Foundation. Obenhaus, Mark, director. Boston, Mass. : Fanlight Productions, 1983. 52 min., color, VHS. Jessica Savitch, narrator.
This gripping and compelling Emmy award-winning documentary follows individuals at an abortion clinic in Chester, Pa. Doctors, nurses, relatives and friends of the patients as well as anti-abortion protestors discuss their views on abortion. In graphic scenes, the film shows two women actually undergoing counseling and a first trimester (suction) abortion.

69. Allen, Doris et al., "Relationships among knowledge, attitudes and behavior of nurses concerning abortion." 81st Annual Convention of the American Psychological Association. 1973. 8: 337-338; bibl.
457 nurses were sent questionnaires asking whether or not they would participate in abortion activities and their actual participation in the past. One usable result is that encouraging abortion is not viewed as an appropriate activity for nurses regardless of individual differences in attitudes towards abortion.

70. Allen, Doris et al. "Factors to consider in staffing an abortion service facility." Journal of Nursing Administration.   4.(July-August 1974): 22-27.
A questionnaire response by 457 nurses in Michigan on their attitudes toward abortion services suggests that when staffing a facility, care should be used to find personnel who are favorably inclined toward abortion.   The data also indicated a need for assessment of the nursing staff's preparation for providing abortion care.

71. American College of Obstetricians and Gynecologists. Standards for Obstetric and Gynecologic Services. 6th ed. Washington, D.C.: ACOG Publications, 1985. 108 p.
"Abortion" section states that ambulatory care facilities should meet the same standards of care as for other surgical procedures.   Abortion in outpatient clinic should be limited to those performed within 14 weeks from the first day of the last menstrual period.   Also recommends exam and laboratory procedures and need to counsel for family planning methods.

72. American Public Health Association.   "Recommended program guide for abortion services." American Journal of Public Health. 63.(1973): 639-644; bibl.
APHA presents a list of guidelines for abortion services following the Supreme Court decision of 1973.   Contains recommendations for education, referral,   counseling, medical care and reporting.

73. Bourne, Judith P. "Abortion: influences on health professionals' attitudes." Hospitals. 46.(July 16, 1972): 80-83.
Attitudes of health professionals toward abortion are affected by four categories of beliefs: 1) basic personality structure and value of the individual 2) kind of involvement the health worker has had with women facing pregnancy or abortion 3) factors that are part of the organization and administration of the abortion service 4) social environment in which the person works.

74. Bozorgi, Nader.   "Termination of pregnancy in a private outpatient clinic." American Journal of Obstetrics and Gynecology.   127.(1977): 763-768; bibl.

A study of 10,890 women who received suction curettage with local anesthesia at a private outpatient clinic showed that complication rates of 6.9 per 1,000 were directly associated with the length of gestation and with the experience of the physicians. The analysis of data suggests that termination of pregnancy in first trimester by suction curettage in a nonhospital setting is a safe operative procedure when high professional standards are maintained.

75. Branch, Benjamin N. "Outpatient termination of pregnancy." In New Concepts in Contraception. eds. Potts, Malcolm and C. Wood. Lancaster, England: Medical and Technical Press, 1972. pp. 175-198.
Views contraceptive choice as a combination of contraception, abortion and sterilization services. The high morbidity and mortality related to classical abortion by untrained personnel can be minimized by new techniques and services. A large proportion of early uncomplicated terminations can be carried out safely without overnight hospitalization and many in independent extramural hospital-affiliated facilities. Contraceptive counseling is an essential part of any abortion-care service.

76. Cates, Willard Jr. "Evaluating the quality of abortion services by measuring outcomes." Advances in Planned Parenthood. 14.(1979): 13; bibl.
Author recommends using outcome measurements as opposed to structural or procedural measurements to determine assessments of the quality of abortion services. Four measurements, physical, psychosocial, physiologic and general are evaluated, along with methodologic problems.

77. Char, Walter F., and McDermott, John F. "Abortions and acute identity crisis in nurses." American Journal of Psychiatry. 128.(February 1972): 952-957;   bibl.
Authors were asked to consult with nurses who worked with abortion patients in three Hawaii hospitals. The nurses suffered significant acute psychological reactions. Resolution of the problems included abreaction, use of psychiatrists as positive therapeutic figures, reestablishment of a more positive identification with patients, regaining objectivity about abortions and realizing the urgent need for a redefinition of the role of the nurse in   abortion services.

78. Danon, Ardis H.   "Organizing an abortion service."   Nursing Outlook. 21.(July, 1973): 460-464.
A nurse involved in setting up an abortion clinic in New York explains how she helped plan, implement procedures, and publicize the clinic.   She also covers the clinic routine and importance of contraceptive counseling.

79. Fairchild, Ellen, and Penfield, A.J.   "Should family planning clinics perform abortions?"   Family Planning Perspectives.   3.(April 1971): 15-17.
Experience in a Syracuse, N.Y. family planning center between July 1, 1970 and March 1, 1971 with 37 first-trimester abortion patients showed that the clinic was quite safe with 4 patients undergoing complications.   Also recommends centers similar to this one handle referrals and contraceptive counseling.

80. Felton, Gerald, and Smith, Roy.   "Administrative guidelines for abortion service."   American Journal of Nursing.   72.(January 1972): 108-109.
Implementation of the abortion law in Hawaii requires guidelines for services so as to make effective use of personnel and best treatment for patients.   Recommends 11 guidelines for staffing, facilities, and kinds of training   programs.

81. Fischer, Edward H., and Caudle, Jan.   "Outsiders' reactions to abortion: personal beliefs and situational influences."   81st Annual Convention of the American Psychological Association.   1973.   8: 339-340; bibl.
198 nursing students were given a test on a hypothetical married woman's desire to have an abortion due to an unintentional pregnancy.   The most striking result was the persistence of beliefs in affecting one's impressions of an abortion client, regardless of conditions peculiar to the case.   Suggests further areas for research would be differential effects of various reasons and circumstances   for abortions and single status.

82. Goldmann, Alice.   "Learning abortion care."   Nursing Outlook.   19.5 (May 1971): 350-352.
Based on a nurse's experience with abortion patients, author recommends more attention be given to nurses' training in family planning and communication skills.   Also recommends conferences be planned before, during and after the students' interaction with abortion patients.

83. Goldsmith, Sadja.   "Early abortion in a family planning clinic."   Family Planning Perspectives.   6.(1974): 119-122; bibl.
Describes integration of early abortion/menstrual induction clinic into family planning clinic.   The ratio of two abortion clinics to eight contraceptive clinics was well accepted by the patients, the medical community and the community at large.   The first year's experience with 560 patients proved that the procedure can be offered at approximately half the cost of hospital abortion, and that a broad range of contraceptive education and counseling can also be provided.

84. Goldstein, Michael S.   "Creating and controlling a medical market: abortion in L.A. after liberalization."   Social Problems. 31.(1984): 514-529;   bibl.
Interviews with physicians performing abortions in Los Angeles in 1982 deals with motives of physicians, group solidarity, stigmatization and sociodemographic variables.   A crucial motive for involvement of the entrepreneurs (100%) and community physicians (71.4%) was an existing social involvement with other physicians.   Entrepreneurs were most likely to specify a positive affinity with the women's movement. [See also his "Abortion as a medical career choice: entrepreneurs, community physicians and others" in   Journal of Health and Social Behavior (25:211-229, 1984)].

85. Hall, Robert E.   "Abortion: physician and hospital attitudes."   American Journal of Public Health.   61.(March 1971): 517-519;   bibl.
In New York State, inconsistent attitudes of physicians regarding abortions and confusing hospital practices (restrictive requirements for abortion patients)has led to the establishment of abortion centers and clinics.   Necessity remains to persuade doctors and hospitals to be more liberal in their treatment of abortion patients.

86. Harper, Mary et al.   "Abortion: do attitudes of nursing personnel affect the patient's perception of care?" Nursing Research.   21.(1972): 327-330; bibl.
A study in attitudes toward abortion of 97 caregivers and of the perceptions of the nursing care they received of 63 abortion patients and 55 nonabortion patients in two Denver hospitals.   The six-month study revealed differences between the two hospital staffs as well as differ-

ences in the patient's perception of nursing care. In the hospital in which staff members viewed abortion less favorably, abortion patients perceived the nursing care as less satisfactory. Nonabortion patients rated the nursing care the same in both hospitals. Authors conclude that a well-planned and well-executed program of in-service education is needed to insure high quality of nursing care in abortion services.

87. Hart, Thomas M., ed. _Abortion in the Clinic and Office Setting._ San Francisco: Society for Humane Abortion, 1972. 105 p.
Proceedings from a symposium on clinic and office abortion procedures on preparing the patient, counseling, medical techniques, legal aspects of abortion and abortion mortality/morbidity statistics.

88. Hausknecht, Richard U. "Free standing abortion clinics: a new phenomenon." _Bulletin of the New York Academy of Sciences._ 49.1 (Nov. 1973): 985-991.
A description of New York City's abortion clinics immediately following the liberalization of the State abortion law makes a distinction between physician-oriented and counselor-oriented clinics. Encourages further establishment of ambulatory abortion facilities.

89. Hendershot, Gerry E., and Grimm, James W. "Abortion attitudes among nurse and social workers." _American Journal of Public Health._ 64.5 (May,1974): 438-441.
A study of training program attendees (social workers, N=419; nurses, N=158) in Tennessee showed that social workers have more liberal attitudes toward abortion than nurses. Authors express concern that because only two-fifths of the nurses approved of most of the abortion requests and fewer than one-fourth approved of abortion on request, nurses might discourage women from having abortions.

90. Hern, Warren M. "Concept of quality care in abortion services." _Advances in Planned Parenthood._ 13.(1978): 63-74; bibl.
Process-oriented questions concerning administrative, medical, and counseling aspects of clinic operation are presented with recommendations. Also provides estimated desirable figures for complication follow-up and contraceptive acceptance rates.

91. Hern, Warren M., and Corrigan, Billie. "What about us? Staff reactions to D & E." Advances in Planned Parenthood 15.(1980): 3-8; bibl.
15 staff members from a small outpatient abortion clinic were polled as to their reactions to first and second trimester D & E procedures. All approved of second trimester abortion in principle, but eight had several reservations. In general, the more direct the physical and visual involvement with D & E the more stress is experienced. Describes coping techniques used by the clinic.

92. Imber, Jonathan B. Abortion and the Private Practice of Medicine. New Haven: Yale University Press, 1986. 164 p.; bibl.
This book is largely based on interviews with 26 ob/gyns between 1978-1982. Chapters 1-2 attempt to clarify abortion as a medical responsibility, while Chapters 3-6 report on the structure of private practice and how physicians reviewed their personal and professional responsibilities towards abortion.

93. Induced Abortion: Guidelines for the Provision of Care and Services. WHO offset publication No.49 . Geneva: World Health Organization, 1979. 69 p.; bibl.
Sets out guidelines for health service administrators who are trying to develop or improve safe and effective clinical services for induced abortion. Discusses services, techniques, training for abortion care, contraceptive counseling and concurrent sterilization.

94. Kane, Francis J. et al. "Emotional reactions in abortion service personnel." Archives of General Psychiatry. 28.409-411(March1973); bibl.
A study of medical personnel at a teaching hospital reports subjective reactions of medical and nursing personnel to the delivery of abortion services. Staff and resident physicians reported occasional depression, anxiety and much obsessive thinking regarding their involvement. Study makes a number of suggestions to improve abortion program in a way so as to minimize emotional distress for staff.

95. Karman, Harvey. "The paramedic abortionist." Clinical Obstetrics and Gynecology. 15.(1972): 379-387; bibl.
A study of 560 terminations performed by volunteer paramedic personnel

supports the hypothesis that carefully selected patients can be aborted safely using nontraumatic techniques in a supervised medical setting.

96. Keith, Louis et al.   "Monitoring care in abortion clinics."   Journal of Reproductive Medicine.   21.(1978): 163-168; bibl.
The responsibility for ensuring high quality outpatient abortion services rests with the clinic medical director.   Three aspects of service must be closely monitored: physician training and selection, patient selection, and abortion outcome monitoring.

97. Kessler, Kenneth, and Weiss, Theodore.   "Ward staff problems with abortions."   International Journal of Psychiatry in Medicine.   5.2 (1974): 97-103;   bibl.
Group sessions with nurses and patients revealed a range of emotions including negative feelings of staff towards patients.   Author recommends including staff in policy planning, minimizing waiting periods for abortions (to avoid saline abortions which were most disturbing to nurses), selecting staff carefully and conducting patient and staff meetings.

98. LoSciuto, Leonard A. et al. "Physicians' attitudes toward abortion." Journal of Reproductive Medicine. 9.(1972): 70-74.
Eight group discussions were held in five areas of the U.S. in an attempt to ascertain physicians' attitudes toward abortion.   Opinion varied widely, with religion, region of the country and size of city of birth being quite important as factors influencing attitudes toward abortion.   Race and sex were not studied, since only one of the physicians was black and only three were women.

99. Maguire, Daniel C.   Reflections of a Catholic Theologian on Visiting an Abortion Clinic.   Washington, D.C.: Catholics for a Free Choice, 1984. 12 p.
Discusses meeting the clinic staff and the women who are waiting for abortions, confronting the picketers, looking at the embryos and reaching conclusions regarding abortion and Catholic theology.

100. Mandel, Mark D.   "An operational and planning staffing model for first

and second trimester abortion services." American Journal of Public Health. 64.8 (August, 1974): 753-764.
New York City's detailed staffing model for both first trimester and second trimester abortion services is outlined. The model assumes a 5-day weekly first and second trimester workload of 30 patients each.

101. Margolis, Alan J. , and Overstreet, E.W. "Legal abortion without hospitalization." Obstetrics and Gynecology. 36.(1970): 479-481.
Proposes that anticipated increase in abortions can be handled by treating patients with pregnancies of no greater than 12 menstrual weeks' duration with an aspiration abortion in an outpatient setting. Reports preliminary experience with 55 outpatients resulted in 8 patients with complications, 2 requiring hospitalization.

102. Mascovich, Paul R. et al. "Attitudes of obstetric and gynecologic residents toward abortion." California Medicine. 119.(August 1973): 29-34; bibl.
48 residents in obstetrics and gynecology in hospitals in San Francisco and Oakland were interviewed about their willingness to perform abortions. Additional questions concerned operational procedures and the physician-patient relationship. Answers revealed that most of the physicians see a social need, but many express boredom and distaste with doing abortions, and ambivalence concerning amniocentesis and abortion for repeaters.

103. McDermott, John F., and Char, Walter F. "Abortion repeal in Hawaii: an unexpected crisis in patient care." American Journal of Orthopsychiatry. 41.4 (1971): 620-626; bibl.
Nurses who worked with abortion patients were found to have great fears of loss of control. Discussion sessions with psychiatrists were aimed at initial ventilation of feelings. Recommends l) nurses be involved in policy making process in order to avoid giving them the feeling of being passive victims of policy; 2) separation of abortion patients from the rest of the obstetric and gynecologic patients.

104. Nathanson, Constance, and Becker, Marshall H. "Obstetricians' attitudes and hospital abortion services." Family Planning Perspectives.

12.1 (February 1980): 26-32;   bibl.
Three variables were studied and analyzed on the abortion services offered
by acute-care general hospitals in Maryland: 1) the hospital's level of
participation in abortion services 2) attitudes of the hospital's obstetrical
staff and community need for services 3)hospital's size and other
organizational dimensions.   Data suggests that the physician's attitudes
are a major factor affecting the number of hospitals at which abortions
are performed and the number of abortions performed.

105. Nathanson, Constance A., and Becker, Marshall H.   "Physician behavior
as a determinant of utilization patterns: the case of abortion."   American
Journal of Public Health.   68.(1978): 1104-1114;   bibl.
Telephone interviews (N=443) and mail questionnaires (N=312) were given
to   ob-gyns in Maryland to determine their abortion practices.   Patient
characteristics have a greater weight in referral decisions than do
physician characteristics.   The decision to refer the patient rather than to
become involved in her case appears most likely when the woman has
insufficient   financial resources to pay for the private case or is a
teenager.   As the authors point out, this is the status of a large proportion
of women who seek   abortions.

106. Nathanson, Constance, and Becker, Marshall H.   "Professional norms,
personal attitudes and medical practice: the case of abortion."   Journal of
Health and Social Behavior.   22.3 (September 1981): 198-211.
A survey of private physicians in one state indicates that physicians with
liberal attitudes towards abortion will offer abortion services regardless
of the normative structure, while conservatively-minded physicians are
dependent on the normative climate.   The majority of conservative
physicians will offer abortion services if the normative climate favors
abortion.

107.   National Abortion Federation.   Standards for Abortion Care.   Rev. ed.
Washington, D.C.. 1986. 17 p.
Contains   obligatory   standards   for   NAF   member   facilities   and
advisory/recommended standards.   Covers ethical aspects, counseling and
informed consent, nursing care, administrative procedures, advertising,
reporting and referral standards.

108. "Nurses' feelings a problem under new abortion law." American Journal of Nursing.   71.2 (February 1971): 350-352.
Comments from a nurses' conference indicate that, even though abortion is legal in New York State, some nurses have hostility towards abortion patients which is reflected in their treatment of the patients.

109. "OB/GYN Nurse Group Takes Stand on Abortion." American Journal of Nursing. 72.7 (July 1972): 1311.
The Nurses Association of the American College of Obstetricians and Gynecologists' statement of "principles and guidelines" on abortion includes sections on responsibilities and ethics for nurses involved in abortion work.

110. Pion, R.J.   "Preventing unwanted pregnancies: role of the hospital." Postgraduate Medicine   51.(January 1972): 172-175;   bibl.
Argues that making a family-planning unit part of the hospital's outreach program will help prevent unwanted pregnancies.

111. Pratt, Gail L. et al. "Connecticut physicians' attitudes toward abortion." American Journal of Public Health. 66(1976): 288-290;   bibl.
Interviews were held with 65 physicians in Connecticut to determine their personal reactions to abortion for 11 hypothetical circumstances under which a woman might request abortion.   Religion, early experiences within the family of orientation and the physician's family of procreation are judged as being far more important as influences on physicians' attitudes to abortion than the broad range of professional experiences which occur later in life.

112. "The RN panel of 500 tells what nurses think about abortion."   R N 33.(June 1970): 40-43.
A scientifically selected cross section of RNs said in response to a questionnaire that 77% are against unrestricted abortion, but favor abortion for certain cases, particularly in rape, incest or defective fetus cases.

113. Roemer, Ruth.   "Equity in abortion services (editorial)."   American

Journal of Public Health. 68.7 (July 1978): 629-631; bibl.
Equity in abortion services has been blocked by geographic factors, limited participation of hospitals, particularly public hospitals and hospitals in rural areas, to provide abortion services. The most serious barrier is the restriction on the use of public funding for abortions sought by indigent women.

114. Rosen, R.A. et al. "Health professionals' attitudes toward abortion." Public Opinion Quarterly. 38.2 (Summer 1974): 159-173.
A nationwide survey on attitudes toward abortion shows that health professionals favor abortion under certain conditions, particularly in order to protect the health of the mother. More than two-thirds of each professional category would help a client obtain a legal abortion under some circumstances. Nursing was the professional group least favorable towards abortion.

115. Schonberg, Leonard A. "Complications of outpatient abortion." Advances in planned parenthood 10.1 (1975): 45-48; bibl.
A survey of 23,290 first-trimester abortions performed at N.Y. City Planned Parenthood centers showed a 6.7% complication rate. Believes low rate due to more rigorous selection of patients and greater experience of the physicians than in hospitals.

116. Schrader, Elinor S. "OR nurses face decision in abortion procedures." AORN Journal 17.13-16; bibl. (May 1973):
Editorial on nurses' role in abortion procedures states that, among other guidelines, nurses have the right to refuse to assist in the performance of abortions and they should not be judgemental when dealing with abortion patients.

117. Seims, Sarah. "Abortion availability in the U.S." Family Planning Perspectives 12.2 (1980): 88-101; bibl.
In 8 out of 10 counties in 1977, no physicians, clinic or hospitals provided abortions. As a result, over one million women were unable to obtain abortion services in their own counties. Recommends program options for meeting these needs.

118. Shelton, James D. et al.   "Abortion utilization: does travel distance matter?" Family Planning Perspectives 8.6 (November/December 1976): 260-261;   bibl.
Analysis of abortion/live birth data in Georgia from 1974-1975 shows that the further the woman must travel in order to obtain an abortion, the less likely she is to get one.   Distance is especially disadvantageous to black teenagers.

119. Siener, Catherine H., and Mahoney, Elizabeth.   "Coordination of outpatient services for patients seeking elective abortion."   Clinical Obstetrics and Gynecology 14.48-59 (March 1971).
Objectives for an abortion service are outlined, as well as the appointment system, clinic procedures, examining and scheduling the patient, family planning instruction and postabortion clinic visit.

120. "A Statement on Abortion by One Hundred Professors of Obstetrics." American Journal of Obstetrics and Gynecology. 112.7 (April 1, 1972): 992-998.
In view of impending legal changes, authors recommend standards for abortion services.   Includes statements that every effort should be made to perform abortions before the end of the first trimester, and that abortions should be made equally available for the rich and the poor. Important summary of changes in professional thinking about abortions.

121. Such-Baer, M.   "Professional staff reaction to abortion work."   Social Casework 55.(1974): 435-441;   bibl.
A survey concerning personal characteristics, attitude toward abortion and emotional reaction to abortion work was taken by doctors, nurses, and social workers in two eastern teaching hospitals.   Social workers are least discomforted by abortion work, possibly because of their identification with the woman and her problems.   Providing physical or medical care and having contact with the aborted fetus correlated with negative emotion on the part of the doctors and nurses.   Suggests implications for social work practice.

122. Swartz, D.P., and Paranjpe, M.K.   "Abortion: medical aspects in a municipal hospital."   Bulletin of the New York Academy of Medicine

47.(August 1971): 845-852;   bibl.
Evaluates abortion services at Harlem Hospital immediately after implementation of the the New York State abortion law, with comparative statistics from the pre-legal period.

123. Tanner, Leonide M. "Developing professional parameters: nursing and social work roles in the care of the induced abortion patient." Clinical Obstetrics and Gynecology14.(December 1972): 1271-1272.
Editor's preface to special section explains that the three articles included examine the abortion patient's need for pre-abortion counseling and assistance, care during hospitalization and follow-up treatment.   Also covers problems in providing care caused by staff attitudes.

124.   "Thirty-three thousand {33,000} doctors speak out on abortion. Modern Medicine (May 14, 1973): 31-35.
64.7% of respondents (N=33,000) to a medical journal questionnaire were in favor of the Supreme Court ruling of 1973.   Doctors in states with large urban centers were most in favor of the ruling, while the lowest approval rate was in the Midwest.   Catholic physicians (52%) had the highest percentage of ethical problems with the ruling.

125.   Walton, Leslie A. et al.   "Development of an abortion service in a large municipal hospital: review of the first year's experience." American Journal of Public Health 64. (January 1974): 77-81; bibl.
Describes an ambulatory abortion service in a municipal hospital.   Among the 6,256 patients there were no deaths, and review of morbidity statistics showed a low rate of complications.   One problem is repeat abortions, despite family planning efforts.   Notes dire need for studies of the psychology and sociology of pregnancy and abortion and the dire need for family planning centers.

126.   Weinstock, Edward et al.   "Abortion needs and services in the United States, 1974-1975." Family Planning Perspectives 8. (1976): 58-69; bibl.
Survey indicates that abortion services are generally concentrated in nonhospital clinics in just one or two metropolitan centers in each state. Data suggests that low-income women, especially those living in outlying areas, are less likely to obtain needed services than the more affluent.

Teenagers, who obtain one-third of all abortions, are still being denied access to abortions by cost, location, or legal factors.

127.   Wolf, Sanford R. et al.   "Assumption of attitudes toward abortion during physician education."   Obstetrics and Gynecology 37.1 (January 1971): 141-147;   bibl.
A questionnaire sent to full-time attending and housestaff members of an ob-gyn department in a teaching hospital revealed there was a neglect of the subject of abortion in medical school curricula.   Specialty education and relationships with obstetric and gynecologic colleagues were the major influences in shaping current attitudes towards abortion.

128.   Wolff, John R.   et al.   "Therapeutic abortion: attitudes of medical personnel leading to complications in patient care.'   American Journal of Obstetrics and Gynecology 110. (1971): 730-733;   bibl.
An early study of records of 50 consecutive patients undergoing therapeutic abortion reveals significant differences in attitudes of the staff.   Both attending staff and residents showed uneasiness and shame in participating in abortions.   Information obtained from a series of seminars points to the conclusion that concern with the issue of death remains paramount.   Authors note that negative feelings of staff need to be resolved before the issue of abortion can be addressed properly.

129.   Women's Research Action Project.   The Abortion Business: A Report on Free-Standing Abortion Clinics.   Rev. ed.   Cambridge, Mass.: Goddard-Cambridge Graduate Program, 1977.   63 p.
Takes a look at a number of clinics in the eastern United States in terms of health care, counseling, conditions of abortion care workers and financial accountability.

130.   Wulff, George J.L., Jr. and Freiman, S.M.   "Elective abortion: complications seen in a free-standing clinic."   Obstetrics and Gynecology 49.3 (March, 1977): 352-357;   bibl.
Of 16,410 elective first trimester abortions performed by Reproductive Health Services of St. Louis, a free-standing clinic, incidence of complications was 1.54%.   The most common complication was incomplete abortion, not apparent until after discharge.   Concludes that it is possible,

with highly trained physicians, to perform first trimester abortions in a clinic setting with satisfactory low incidence of complications.

131. Yaloff, Beverly et al. "Nursing care in an abortion unit." Clinical Obstetrics and Gynecology 14.(March 1971): 67-80.
Describes all details of nursing care in the abortion unit at The New York Hospital, including admissions, preoperative and post-abortion care and medical   techniques.

132. Young, Philip E.   "Abortion and menstrual extraction for the ambulatory patient." Clinical Obstetric & Gynecology 17.3 (September 1974): 277-290;   bibl.
In view of recent (1973) changes in the abortion law, reviews standards for ambulatory abortion care, acceptable level of complications, possible long-term complications, specific protocols for menstrual extraction in the office and   ambulatory in-hospital abortions.

3

Abortion Decision

133. <u>Abortion: Listen to the Woman</u>.   Planned Parenthood of Los Angeles. 1985. Audiocassette,   50 minutes.
Professor Daniel Maguire discusses the abortion decision as only part of a larger world situation.   States that the woman should not be blamed for the decision and that instead society should go after the multiple causes which create unwanted pregnancies.   Relates the decision to sexism, military budget, and poverty.   As a prescription for dealing with abortion in the future, we need "imagination, anger, courage and mirth."

134. Allgeier, A.R. et al.   "Response to requests for abortion: the influence of guilt and knowledge." <u>Journal of Applied Social Psychology</u> 12.4   (July-August 1982): 281-291; bibl.
Participants (who varied in their levels of sex guilt and sex knowledge) from an introductory psychology class were asked to read case histories of women applying for abortion.   The case histories varied so that the pregnancy was due to either failure of the contraceptive or failure of the person to use the contraceptive consistently.   Low sex guilt participants were more favorable towards abortion requests than were high sex guilt participants, but both groups were more favorable towards abortion because of a contraceptive method failure than a failure to use contraceptives consistently.

135. Ashton, J.R.   "Components of delay amongst women obtaining termination of pregnancy." <u>Journal of Biosocial Science</u> 12.3 (July 1980): 261-273;   bibl.
A study of delay among a group of women in England shows the impor-

tance of age. Only 47% of women aged 17-18 years obtained their abortion before 12 weeks gestation compared with more than 70% of women of other age groups.

136. Ashton, J.R.   "Patterns of discussion and decision-making amongst abortion patients."   Journal of Biosocial Science   12.3 (June 1980): 247-259;   bibl.
Discussion and decision-making patterns among a group of women at two centers in England who had already made abortion decisions showed that "significant others" played a major role in the decision process, and that, with the exception of family doctors and pregnancy counselors, professional staff members are involve in discussion after the abortion decision is made.

137. Barr, Samuel J. with Dan Abelow.   A Woman's Choice.   New York: Rawson Associates Pub., Inc. , 1977 (reprinted 1979, Public Information Press). 306 p.
Dr. Barr, a gynecologist who also owns an abortion clinic, provides accounts of his patients.   Barr stresses the importance of counseling and birth control, while affirming that the decision to abort is a serious one on the part of the woman and her doctor.

138. Blumenfield, Michael.   "Psychological factors involved in request for elective abortion."   Journal of Clinical Psychiatry.   39.1 (January 1978): 17-25;   bibl.
A study of 13 first abortion and 13 repeat abortion patients demonstrated that the failure of contraception was not because women did not have access to   adequate contraception.   In 9 of 26 patients the data suggests that the women had an underlying conflictual wish to become pregnant.

139. Bracken, Michael B.   et al.   "Abortion, adoption or motherhood: an empirical study of decision-making during pregnancy."   American Journal of Obstetrics and Gynecology 130.(February I, I978): 151-262.
A detailed study of 249 single women examines why some women with almost identical sociodemographic profiles choose to deliver while others choose to abort.   In this population (young, three-quarters black,

one-third pregnant for the first time, and two-thirds on welfare), the decision seemed to be based on circumstances surrounding the particular pregnancy rather than the characteristics of the mothers.   Adoption is not an option in this particular population group.

140. Bracken, Michael B. et al. "The decision to abort and psychological sequelae." Journal of Nervous and Mental Disease 158.(1974): 154-162; bibl.
A brief critique of the psychological literature on abortion emphasizes the need to consider the decision-making process and the psychological and sociocultural milieu in which the decision was made. A sample of 489 women from a New York abortion clinic demonstrated that reaction among older women was significantly more favorable when the partner supported the decision. Among younger women, parental support was more important for a favorable reaction.

141. Bracken, Michael B. An Epidemiological Study of Psychosocial Correlates of Delayed Decisions to Abort. New Haven: Yale University, 1974.
Study of women in New Haven and New York demonstrates that women delaying abortion were significantly more likely to be black, young, single and pregnant by a boyfriend. Factors associated with delay in New York but not New Haven women included: absence of support from significant others, more people knowing about the abortion, pregnancy denial, no previous induced abortion, low coital rates and poor contraception.

142. Bracken, Michael B., and Kasl, Stanislav V. "First and repeat abortions: a study of decision- making and delay." Journal of Biosocial Science 7.(1975): 473-491; bibl.
In a sample of women undergoing abortion at a N.Y. clinic, women having a repeat procedure had delayed significantly less in seeking abortion than had first-time patients. Psychological reactions to the decision did not differ between women having first and repeat abortions.

143. Bracken, Michael, and Swigar, Mary E. "Factors associated with delay in seeking induced abortion." American Journal of Obstetrics and

Gynecology 113.(1972): 301-309; bibl.
443 women requesting abortion at the Yale-New Haven Hospital were interviewed.   Authors analyze data with the stage of pregnancy at the time of interview as the dependent variable.   Women between 11-20 weeks of pregnancy were significantly more likely to be under 21 years old, single, have 0 or 1 living child, be black, not finished high school, and Protestant.   Authors caution that data will vary from hospital to hospital, and recommends other studies be carried out, in particular of the decision-making process and also of the factors within the medical care system which might lead to delay in seeking abortion.

144. Brewer, Colin.   "Induced abortion after feeling fetal movements: its causes and emotional consequences."   Journal of Biosocial Science 10.2 (April 1978): 203-208;   bibl.
Study of 40 women who had abortions between 20 and 24 weeks gestation and had felt fetal movements showed a wide range of causes for late abortion.   Menstrual irregularities and misdiagnosis were common.   There was little evidence of psychopathology.   The emotional consequences of abortion after quickening seem to be less important than has been suggested.

145. Brewer, Colin.   "Third time unlucky: a study of women who have had three or more legal abortions."   Journal of Biosocial Science 9.(1977): 99-105;   bibl.
Of 50 English women who were having their third or subsequent legal abortion, 23 were pregnant because their contraceptive method had failed, 24 because of erratic contraceptive use and 3 because they had changed their mind about the pregnancy.   There was no evidence of abortion being used as a method of birth control.

146. Burr, Winthrop A., and Schulz, Kenneth F.   "Delayed abortion in an area of easy accessibility."   JAMA 244.1 (July 4, 1980): 44-48; bibl.
Examined potential correlates of late abortion in a study of 1,066 women at two Washington, D.C. clinics.   A history of irregular periods is the strongest single determinant for seeking a late abortion.   There was also evidence of psychological maturity and moral quandry as contributors to abortion delay.   Suggests that the problem of late abortions is not necessarily one which can be influenced by public health interventions.

147. Cornelio, David A. A Descriptive Study of the Attitudes of Males Involved in Abortion. New York: Columbia University Teachers College, 1983.
Interviews with sixty males involved in abortion decisions revealed that they want and need to take part in decisions regarding abortion. Most males in the study felt that both partners should bear equal responsibility for the pregnancy and in deciding on the abortion. There was a strong correlation between males who spoke positively about the abortion and those who said they had much verbal communication with their partners about abortion.

148. Crabtree, Pamela Hinckley. Personality Correlates of the Delayed Abortion Decision. Garden City, New York: Adelphi University, 1980.
Results of study of 80 women, 40 of whom were 6-12 weeks pregnant and 40 of whom were I6-24 weeks pregnant. Data analysis confirmed the thesis that late abortion patients differ substantially from early abortees in their psychological reaction to pregnancy and abortion. Late abortions reported more external influence in their decision-making process and more recent behavioral changes.

149. Diamond, Milton et al. "Sexuality, birth control and abortion: a decision-making sequence." Journal of Biosocial Science. 5.(1973): 347-361.
Data and commentary from the Hawaii Pregnancy , Birth Control, and Abortion Study. Presents behavioral and contraceptive correlates of women from a special population pool referred to as a contraceptive cohort. Findings indicate that coitus was anticipated by the majority of women, but pregnancy was unplanned. Regardless of whether pregnancy was planned or unplanned, one woman in three chose abortion. Marital status, age, and religion affected the decision as to whether or not to have an abortion.

150. Eisen, Marvin, and Zellman, Gail L. "Factors predicting pregnancy resolution decision satisfaction of unmarried adolescents." Journal of Genetic Psychology. 145.2 (December, 1984): 231-239; bibl.
Among 297 pregnant, unmarried teenagers interviewed 6 months after delivery or abortion, 82% said they would make the same decision as they had made initially. Among the abortion group, two measures of initial

abortion attitudes--approval of abortion for herself and general attitudes towards abortion--are associated with postdecision satisfaction. { For an expanded version of this paper, see Genetic Psychology Monographs August 1983 v. 108 (1) 69-95}.

151. Fielding, W.L. et al. "Comparison of women seeking early and late abortion." American Journal of Obstetrics and Gynecology 131.(1978): 304-310; bibl.
Differential characteristics of 697 women desiring induced abortion were studied. Those with greatest delay in seeking abortion tended to be young, unmarried and minimally educated. Contributing factors of denial, ambivalence, fear and previous menstrual irregularity accounted for two thirds of the cases. Suggests community social service and educational efforts should be aimed at teaching the population most at risk from delayed abortion.

152. Four Young Women. Schwarz, Leonard C., producer. Espar, David, and Schwarz, Leonard C., directors. Palo Alto: Veriation Films, 1973. 20 min.; color, VHS.
Documentary about four different young women and how they made their abortion decisions. One woman and her partner planned to marry, but not right away. Another woman married her partner and had the baby, but had a later abortion when she became pregnant 5 months after the baby was born. Two single women without partners talk about how the decision affected themselves and their family. At the end of the tape, a doctor explains two abortion techniques.

153. Freeman, Ellen W. "Abortion:subjective attitudes and feelings." Family Planning Perspectives 10.(May/June 1978): 150-155; bibl.
A study of 329 women pre-abortion and 106 women post-abortion shows that abortion is not an idiosyncratic choice by a few atypical women but is undergone by average women who are neither independent and individualistic nor emotionally disturbed. Author concludes that abortion was a difficult decision and that the women had not acted consistently to prevent contraception, but that contraceptive behavior was strikingly more effective and consistent in the post-abortion period.

154. Freeman, Ellen W. et al. "Emotional distress patterns among women having first or repeat abortions." Obstetrics and Gynecology 55.(May 1980): 630-636; bibl.
Pre-abortion and post-abortion emotional distress factors and associated demographic characteristics were compared for women having first abortions and those having repeat abortions. Prior to abortion, elevated distress levels were similar in both groups. After abortion, repeat aborters continued to have significantly higher emotional distress scores in interpersonal relationships.

155. Friedlander, Myrna L. et al. "Abortion: predicting the complexity of the decision-making process." Women & Health 9.1 (Spring 1984): 43-54; bibl.
Reviews and evaluates literature on decision-making in abortion. Reports on results of questionnaire administered to women attending a clinic to obtain 1st trimester abortions (N=291). The abortion decision was significantly more complex with a lengthier and more stable relationship with the sexual partner and when he was consulted, and when employment was less salient to the individual.

156. Gibb, Gerald D.   "A comparative study of recidivists and contraceptors along the dimensions of locus of control and impulsivity." International Journal of Psychology 19.6 (December 1984): 581-591. Research effort was aimed at determining if differences exist between contraceptors and recidivists with respect to locus of control and impulsivity. Repeat aborters undergoing abortions and nulliparas seeking contraceptive services scored significantly lower on impulsivity tests than initial and repeat aborters seeking contraceptive services. No differences were found between groups with respect to locus of control.

157. Gibb, Gerald D., and Millard, Richard J. "Research on repeated abortion: state of the field: 1973-1979." Psychological Reports 48.2 (April 1981): 415-424; bibl.
A review of the literature on repeated abortion indicates that the U.S. may soon approach the recidivism rates already found in Asian and European women. Research needs to resolve the "contra-ceptor/contraceptive failure controversy." In addition, authors recommend researchers look at per aborters and establish a medical

record linkage system to permit accurate reporting of abortion statistics.

158. Gilligan, Carol et al.   "A naturalistic study of abortion decisions." In   Selman, Robert L. et al., eds.   Clinical-Developmental Psychology, pp. 69-90; bibl.   San Francisco: Jossey-Bass, l980.
A study of 24 women who had been referred through pregnancy counseling services or abortion clinics.   Discrepancies between hypothetical judgements and reasoning about an actual choice can predict the clinical outcome of crisis.

159. Group for the Advancement of Psychiatry.   Committee on Psychiatry and the Law. The Right to Abortion: A Psychiatric View.   New York : Charles Scribners' Sons, 1970.
An important position statement by the GAP Committee on Psychiatry and the Law recommending that abortion be entirely removed from the domain of criminal law. As psychiatrists, the group recommends physician explore with the pregnant woman the basis of her motivation, so as to clarify impulsive, manipulative or self-destructive elements in the decision to abort.

160. Howe, Barbara et al.   "Repeat abortions: blaming the victims." American   Journal of Public Health   69.(1979): 1242-1246; bibl.
A study of 1505 women from an abortion clinic revealed that 16.9% were repeaters, almost identical to the national average for 1975.   Both first time and repeaters reject the premise that abortion is a primary or even back-up birth control method.   Nearly one-half of the abortion repeaters who were not contracepting were unable or fearful of using the most effective methods of contraception.   See also letter criticizing study and response by authors (AJPH v. 70(6), June 1980 p. 637).

161. Jacobssen, L.B. et al.   "Repeat aborters--first aborters: a social psychiatric comparison." Social Psychiatry 11.(1976): 75-86; bibl.
In a Swedish study, 45 women with repeat abortions and 92 women seeking their first abortion were examined.   The repeat aborters had more children, were more often employed outside the home, had more

sexual partners and had a greater experience of contraceptives.

162. Jekel, James F. et al. "Induced abortion and sterilization among women who became mothers as adolescents." _American Journal of Public Health_ 67.(1977): 621-625; bibl.
Four cohorts of urban women who delivered before age 18 were followed for several periods (from 6-12 years) to determine use of abortion and sterilization.   Approximately 40% of all four groups used either abortion or sterilization, or occasionally both, to control subsequent fertility. The heavy reliance on surgical means of fertility control was not anticipated.   Results raise a number of questions regarding fertility control needs.

163. Johnstone, F.D., and Vincent, L. "Factors affecting gestational age at termination of pregnancy." _Lancet_ 1 (September 29, 1973): 717-719; bibl.
A study of 372 patients at the Chelsea Hospital for Women in London demonstrates that patients presenting late differed in social and demographic factors from those presenting early in pregnancy.   Where the interval was longer, the women was more likely to be 21 or younger, to be single, to have had no children or one child only, and to have no means of support.   While there were psychological reasons why many women had late abortions, most of the delay occurred because of problems in the medical care system.

164. Joseph, Carol. "Factors related to delay for legal abortions performed at a gestational age of 20 weeks or more." _Journal of Biosocial Science_ 17.3 (July 1985): 327-337; bibl.
Between 1981-1982 the Royal College of Obstetricians and Gynaecologists undertook a national survey of late abortion practice in England and Wales.   Delay in recognizing the pregnancy, either by the woman or her doctor, was reported as one of the reasons for delay in 38.5% of the women.   The doctors attributed 84% of the delay in the private sector and 79% in the National Health Service to the women themselves.

165. Kaltreider, Nancy B. "Emotional patterns related to delay in

decision to seek legal abortion: a pilot study."   California Medicine
118.(May,1978):   23-27; bibl.
A pilot study of 18 women who underwent first trimester abortion or
second trimester abortion reveals that the women in the second
trimester group had poor self-images and more disturbed relationships
with their parents than did the first trimester group.   After the
abortion, the first trimester group focused on a sense of relief while the
second trimester women expressed mixed feelings or tried to cope by
denial.

166. Kaltreider, Nancy B.   "Psychological factors in mid-trimester
abortion."   International Journal of Psychiatry in Medicine 4.2 (Spring,
1973): 125-134.
A comparative psychiatric evaluation of 18 women with similar
backgrounds suggests that the delay of the abortion decision until second
trimester involves multiple psychological factors.   The eight women who
presented late had a pattern of disturbed parental relationships, reliance
on denial as a defense mechanism, and ambivalence towards the
pregnancy.

167. Kerenyi, Thomas D. et al.   "Reasons for delayed abortion: results of
four hundred interviews."   American Journal of Obstetrics and Gynecology
117.(1973): 299-311; bibl.
Study compares 200 patients requiring late abortion and 200 patients
requesting early abortion in an attempt to discover reasons for delaying
abortion.   Questionnaire covered patients' demographic background, facts
related to pregnancies, contraceptive practices and sexual attitudes and
behavior.   The reasons causing the delay were attributable to the health
care system in 1 in 4 patients.   Environmental factors and certain
manifestations of personality structure appeared to be responsible in the
rest of the late group. Lack of basic sexual education is a major
contributing factor to late abortions, and authors suggest physicians
become more involved in referring patients to counseling.

168. Leach, Judith.   "The repeat abortion patient."   Family Planning
Perspectives 9.1 (January/February 1977): 37-39; bibl.
A study of repeat abortion patients revealed that they are more often
dissatisfied with themselves, perceive themselves as victims of bad

luck, and express negative feelings about themselves more frequently than do women who are obtaining abortions for the first time.

169. Lincoln, Elizabeth. _A Case Study of the Reproductive Experience of Women Who Have Had Three or More Induced Abortions_. University of Pittsburgh, 1982.
Information from eight women who had three or more induced abortions since 1973 was analyzed to see if any common themes emerged from the group and what similarities there were with the literature on repeat abortions. The participants felt out of control in regard to the pregnancies, had a conservative sex role, feared health effects and had problematic relationships with partners.

170. Luker, Kristin. _Abortion and the Decision Not to Contracept._ Berkeley, Ca. : University of California Press, 1975. 207 p.; bibl.
Based on information obtained from a survey of medical records of 500 women as well as in-depth interviews with 50 women, all of whom sought abortions at a San Francisco clinic. This book reconstructs scenarios of contraceptive risk taking which leads to unwanted pregnancies. Luker theorizes that not all women who seek abortions are neurotic and irrational. Instead, their decisions must be viewed in context with their sexual relationships and external pressures.

171. Luscutoff, Sidney A., and Elms, Alan C. "Advice in the abortion decision." _Journal of Counseling Psychology_ 22.2 (March 1975): 140-146; bibl.
Subjects (224 abortion patients, 71 obstetrics patients and 101 nonhospitalized controls) were asked to report the number of contacts for advice they had made when forming pregnancy or non-pregnancy related decisions. Abortion subjects reported a mean of 3.01 contacts (versus 4.94 per obstetrics patient and 5.04 per nonpregnant subject).

172. Mace, David R. _Abortion: the Agonizing Decision_. Nashville: Abingdon Press, 1972. 144 p.; bibl.
A general book on non-biased abortion counseling by a medical school professor. Contains chapter "The world within the womb" which explains development of the fetus and how pregnancy can be terminated. Also

deals with the need to make abortion an "informed decision" so the woman can be psychologically at ease afterwards.

173. Maguire, Marjorie J., and Maguire, Daniel C. _Abortion: A Guide to Making Ethical Choices_.   Washington, D.C.: Catholics for a Free Choice, 1983. 44 p.
In the form of questions and answers, this guide explores various issues related to abortion from a Catholic viewpoint to help the woman facing the decision develop criteria for ethical decision-making.

174. Mallory, George B. et al.   "Factors responsible for delay in obtaining interruption of pregnancy."   _Obstetrics and Gynecology_ 40.(1972): 556-562;   bibl.
To explore factors which lead women to obtain abortions after the 12th week,a representative sample of women undergoing early (suction curettage) and late (saline instillation) were interviewed.   Women having a late abortion were more likely to be younger, single, and nulliparous, and less likely to have ever used contraception than were women having early abortions.   Of patients undergoing late abortion, 55% were delayed for personal reasons while 26% were delayed for reasons attributable to the health care system.   Suggests that decreasing the percentage of late abortions will require improvement in the availability of early abortions but also in intensive health education and counseling.

175. Muhr, Janice Ruth.   _Psychological Adjustment to First Trimester Abortion_.   Evanston, Illinois: Northwestern University, 1978.   327 p.
A study of the processes by which women make abortion decisions. Based on a survey of women at an urban abortion clinic, the study indicates that a woman's experience with abortion is affected by her handling of conflicting social, interpersonal, and personal meanings attached to pregnancy and abortion.

176. "My Conscience Speaks: Catholic Women Discuss their Abortions." Abortion in Good Faith series. Washington, D.C.: Catholics for a Free Choice, 1981. 48 p.
Eight Catholic women of Black, Irish, Italian, Puerto Rican and Slavic origins tell about their abortions, both legal and illegal.

177. Pearson, J.F.   "Pilot study of single women requesting a legal abortion." Journal of Biosocial Science 3.(October 1971): 417-448; bibl. In depth interviews with eleven unmarried women in London are recorded. Observations from the study indicated that knowledge and motivation were individual factors that could not account exclusively for the women becoming pregnant.

178. Personal Decisions. Goodwin, Tom, and Wurzburg, Geraldine, producers. Wiedenmayer, Joseph, editor.   Planned Parenthood Federation of America, Inc., distributed by The Cinema Guild, 1985. 28 min., color, VHS.
A number of women, of varying ages and in varying socioeconomic circumstances, tell about the abortion decision.   Dr. Kenneth Edelin stresses the indignities and medical hazards of illegal abortions and notes the obligation of the medical profession to help women have safe abortions.   Partners and parents of women who have made the abortion decision talk about their feelings about the abortion.

179. Poliak, Jose, and Morgenthau, Joan E. "Adolescent aborters: factors associated with gestational age." New York State Journal of Medicine 82.2 (February 1982): 176-179; bibl.
A study of differential characteristics of 113 pregnant teenagers seeking abortion showed that teenagers 13-16 are significantly more likely to terminate pregnancy after 11 weeks than the 17-20 age group. Teenagers aborting after 11 weeks are also significantly more likely to have never used any form of contraception than those aborting earlier.

180.   Robins, Sharon, and Granger, Bruce. Having a Wonderful Abortion. New York: Exposition Press, 1971. 152 p.
A first-hand account of a Canadian woman undergoing a legal abortion in London, England.

181.   Rosen, Raye Hudson and Martindale, Lois J.   "Abortion as 'deviance'--traditional female roles vs. the feminine perspective." Social Psychiatry 15. (1980): 193-208; bibl.
A questionnaire given to a sample of women from a study of decision-

making on unplanned pregnancies evaluated perceived competence and female role orientation.   Only 4% of the aborters and 3% of those who chose to keep the child said that someone else had primary responsibility for the decision.   The aborters indicated a less traditional orientation to the female role than did those who kept the child, but saw themselves as competent, self-directed, legitimately sexual persons.   {See also his 1978 article, "Sex role perceptions and the abortion decision in Journal of Sex Research (Nov. 1978, 14(4)231-245}.

182. Ryan, Ione J., and Dunn, Patricia C.   "College students' attitudes toward shared responsibility in decisions about abortion: implications for counseling."   Journal of American College Health 31.6 (June 1983): 231-235;   bibl.
A survey of college students' perceptions of the extent to which males should be involved in abortion decision making revealed that both male and female college students are in favor of shared responsiblity in abortion decision making.   The male students indicate a greater willingness to assume more responsibility for an abortion decision in casual sexual situations than female students would   allow.

183. Schneider, Sandra M. et al.   "Repeat aborters."   American Journal of Obstetrics and Gynecology 126.3 (October 1, 1976): 316-320;   bibl.
116 women seeking a repeat abortion were compared with three groups of women not seeking a repeat abortion but otherwise similar.   Women who have had an abortion increase their use of contraception thereafter and remain more likely to use it than first abortion women.   However, such contraception is less than that of sexually active women.

184. Shaw, Paul C.   "An investigation of the abortion decision process." Psychology: A Quarterly Journal of Human Behavior   16.2 (Summer 1979): 11-19.
Analysis of a questionnaire given to 195 women who had abortions indicated that many women were motivated by personal, pragmatic considerations, including factors related to financial, educational or career goals.   Influence of the sexual partner seems to be an important source of support in the abortion   decision.

185. Shepard, Mary Jo, and Bracken, Michael B. "Contraceptive practice and repeat induced abortion: an epidemiological investigation." Journal of Biosocial Science 11.3 (July 1979): 289-302; bibl.
The relationship between abortion experience and contraceptive practice is examined among women having a repeat or first abortion (N=443). A previous abortion was the single most important predictor of past contraceptive practices. Also studies sociodemographic associations for the group.

186. Smetana, Judith G. Concepts of Self and Morality: Women's Reasoning about Abortion. New York: Praeger Publishers, 1982. 168 p.
Based on a dissertation at the University of California at Santa Cruz, this work explores social reasoning and how decisions are made about abortion. The decision to continue or terminate an unwanted pregnancy is discussed not as an isolated choice but rather in relation to the ways individuals conceptualize and act upon the social world. Deals with social-cognititive development and   psychological perspectives on abortion.

187. Steinhoff, Patricia G. et al. "Women who obtain repeat abortions: a study based on record linkage." Family Planning Perspectives 11.(1979): 30-38;   bibl.
A record linkage study of repeat abortions in Hawaii finds no evidence that women are substituting abortion for contraception. Repeat abortion accounts for approximately one half of subsequent pregnancy experience within five years after a first induced abortion.

188. Tietze, Christopher. "Human rights in relationship to induced abortion." Journal of Sex Research 10.2 (May 1974): 89-96.
In a speech, Dr. Tietze poses and answers questions regarding the rights of the fetus and patient and who has the decision-making authority. Although other persons may give counsel, the final decision should rest with the pregnant woman, and the professionals should then give her full support.

189. Tietze, Christopher. "The "problem" of repeat abortions." Family Planning Perspectives 6.3 (Summer 1974): 148-150; bibl.
Although reliable information on the frequency of repeat legal abortions is not yet (1974) available, Tietze predicts that a significant incidence of

repeat abortions can be expected within a year or two following a first abortion or liberalization of the abortion law.   Estimates of expected repeat abortions lend support to the need for skillful counseling and postabortion contraception.

190. Tietze, Christopher.   "Repeat abortion--why more?"   Family Planning Perspectives 10.(1978): 286-288;   bibl.
The risk of repeat abortion for women who have already had one abortion is much greater than the risk of first abortion because of the age distributions of the women, sexual activity of the repeat aborters and fertility.

191. Weisheit, Eldon.   Should I Have an Abortion?   St. Louis: Concordia Publishing House, 1976. 101 p.
Discusses a woman's options during an unwanted pregnancy and looks at different ways of approaching the pregnancy, including abortion.   Written from a Christian, non-judgemental point of view.

192. Women Who Have Had an Abortion. Martha Stuart Communications, Inc. 1972. 29 min.; color; 3/4" U-matic video cassette.
A group of women, all of whom have had at least one abortion, informally discuss their experiences and how they made the abortion decision.
Several individuals talk about having babies and how it affected them in contrast to their abortions.   In answer to the discussion leader's question on what would be a "perfect abortion clinic," the women respond with "free," "on demand," "warm," "personal," and "in the community."

4

Abortion Techniques
(General)

193. The Abortion Experience. Ellis, Nadene, producer. Miller, David, director. SAP Productions, 1985. 28 min., color, VHS. Hosted by Veryl Rosenbaum.
A short film dealing with the physical and emotional aspects of abortion. Several women tell what they felt were negative or positive aspects about their abortions. One segment has a physician in a clinic room explaining techniques used in early (suction) abortion, showing equipment, laminaria, dilators, cannulae and the suction machine. He also discusses possible pain, use of anesthesia and what to look for in terms of complications. Film does not cover mid or late trimester problems or medical techniques.

194. Benditt, John. "Second trimester abortion in the United States." Family Planning Perspectives 11.(Nov/Dec. 1979): 358-361.
Reports results of a conference on second trimester abortion held in Chapel Hill, N.C. Two major trends were noted since the 1973 Supreme Court decision: a sharp reduction in mortality from second trimester abortions and the replacement of saline instillation by D & E as the most widely used second trimester technique. Concerns which still need to be addressed: long-term effects on future childbearing; factors which cause women to delay the abortion decision; methods to reduce the number of late abortions.

195. Berger, G.S. et al., editors. Second Trimester Abortion. September 27-28, 1979. Boston: John Wright/PSG Inc., 1981. 340 p.; bibl.

Thorough examination of all aspects of second trimester abortion, including socioeconomic factors, methods for inducing termination, morbidity and mortality, future reproduction and psychological factors. Concludes with evaluations of the future of second trimester abortion in the U.S. and world and ways of preventing the need for second trimester abortions.

196. Bluett, Desmond G.   "A review of one thousand uncomplicated vaginal operations for abortion." Contraception 7.1 (1973): 11-25; bibl.
Of 1,000 patients undergoing abortion, all at an outpatient clinic in England, 7.8% received abortions up to the 9th week of gestation, 77.2% between the 9th-12th week of gestation, and 15% between the 13th-16th week of gestation. There were no complications resulting from the D & C method. Compares his study results with 6 other recent major studies reported in the literature. Concludes that low morbidity in current study may result from outpatient setting and performance of the abortion under short general anesthesia.

197. Brenner, William E.   "Second trimester interruption of pregnancy." In Progress in gynecology, v. 6.   eds. Taymor, Melvin L., and Green, Thomas H.   New York: Grune & Stratton, 1975. pp. 421-444; bibl.
Reviews current (1975) research on second trimester abortion, discussing minor and major surgical procedures and extraovular administration of intrauterine solutions.

198. Burnett, L.S. et al.   "Evaluation of abortion: techniques and protocols." Hospital Practice 10.8 (August 1975): 97-105; bibl.
Authors review current abortion protocols and recommend that special units (separate from other OB/GYN facilities) are needed for maximum safety and efficiency.   They also review techniques and state that prostaglandins and their analogues need to be investigated further to increase their utility.

199. Burnett, L.S. et al. "Techniques of pregnancy termination, Pt. II." Obstetrical and Gynecological Survey 29.(1974): 6-42; bibl.
{See Wentz, Anne for Part I of this article}. A concise summary of the techniques of pregnancy termination for mid-trimester abortions.

Concludes that there does not exist a self-administered agent effective in termination of both first and second trimester pregnancies. The only successful attempt to improve vacuum evacuation has been the development of vacuum curettage, while the use of prostaglandins needs more clinical trials.

200. Chaudry, Susan L. et al. Pregnancy Termination in Midtrimester--Review of Major Methods. Population Information Program: Population Reports Series F . Washington, D.C.: The George Washington University Medical Center, September, 1976. 16 p.; bibl.
Reviews techniques and literature of the four midtrimester abortion methods: surgical evacuation, intrauterine injection of solutions, intrauterine insertion of devices, and extrauterine methods. Contains excellent tables comparing selected studies (1973-1975) on the various methods.

201. Corson, Stephen L. et al. Fertility Control.   Boston: Little, Brown and Company, 1985. 344 p.; bibl.
Text covering various aspects of fertility regulation, including surgical methods, hormonal methods, barriers and vaginal chemical agents, intrauterine contraception and other methods.   Surgical methods section contains chapters on   first and mid-trimester abortion technology.

202. The Diagram Group. Woman's Body: An Owner's Manual. New York: Paddington Press, 1977. 431 p.
Section "Methods of Abortion" gives clear diagrams and concise statements of techniques.

203. Eclipse of Reason.   Bernard N. Nathanson, M.D., Executive Producer. R. Anderson, Director.   Bernadell, Inc., 1987. Introduced by Charlton Heston and narrated by Bernard Nathanson. 27 min.; color; VHS.
Updates "Silent Scream" (1977).   Concentrates on late (2nd-3rd trimester) abortions. Films a physician performing late abortion using D & E technique.   Shows view of fetus through fetascope.   Contains commentary by physicians opposed to abortions and two women who underwent abortions, one with physical complications and the other with psychological complications.

204. Federation of Feminist Women's Health Centers. <u>A New View of a Woman's Body</u>. New York: Simon & Schuster, 1981. 174 p.
"Menstrual extraction" demonstrates with diagrams and line drawings how the technique can be done at home or in a self-help group. "Feminist abortion care" demonstrates various abortion techniques.

205. Fleming, Alice. <u>Contraception, Abortion, Pregnancy.</u> Nashville: Thomas Nelson Inc., 1974. 92 p.
A concise and clear account of contraception and medical techniques of abortion.

206. Hern, Warren M. "Midtrimester abortion." <u>Obstetrics and Gynecology Annual</u> 10.(1981): 375-422; bibl.
Reviews literature on the subject of medical techniques for midtrimester abortion. Explains in detail various abortion techniques by type of operation and also by fetal age. Also analyzes management of complications, recovery, and follow-up, postoperative medications and postabortion contraception.

207. King, Theodore M. et al. "Abortion: practice and promise." <u>Advances in Planned Parenthood</u> 10.(1975): 204-214; bibl.
Documents literature written during the 1970-1975 period. The most impressive development has been the evolution of abortion techniques, particularly the use of suction curettage for first-trimester abortions. Concurrent with the recognition of the unsuitability of surgery for midtrimester abortion, the life-threatening sequelae associated with hypertonic saline were appreciated. This led to the acceptance of the prostaglandin F2alpha. States there is need for well-constructed studies on late sequelae of induced abortion.

208. Margolis, Alan J., and Goldsmith, Sadja. "First-trimester induced abortion." In <u>Progress in Gynecology, v. 6</u>, eds. Taymor, Melvin L., and Green, Thomas H. New York: Grune & Stratton, 1975. pp. 401-419; bibl.
Reviews current (1975) research on first trimester abortion, including the development of the uterine aspiration technique. Discusses setting and procedures for evaluation of patient before and after abortion.

209. Neubardt, Selig, and Schulman, Harold. <u>Techniques of Abortion.</u> 2nd ed.   Boston: Little, Brown and Company, 1977.   163 p.; bibl.
An excellent summary of abortion techniques.   Includes chapters on creating an abortion service and on contraception, plus a personal essay by Neubardt on his observation of Japanese abortion techniques, primarily the use of laminaria.

210. <u>Physiology of Miscarriage and Abortion</u>. Inner Woman series.   Bob Lipson, Director.   Jeanne Findlater, Producer.   28 min., Film. Detroit: WXYZ, 1975. guide included; 3 p., bibl.
Marilyn Poland, R.N., and David I. Lipschutz, M.D. talk about spontaneous abortion (miscarriage) and induced abortion. Covers techniques, possible complications, implications for future pregnancies, how women feel afterwards and risks of illegal abortions.

211. Pion, R.J. "Evaluation of Abortion Techniques." In <u>Regulation of Human Fertility.</u> eds. Evans, T.N., and Moghissi, K.S.   Detroit: Wayne State University Press, 1976. pp. 164-173; bibl.
Reviews findings and experiences from the Hawaii Pregnancy, Birth Control and Abortion Study (PBCA). Discusses methods of early and late abortion and menstrual aspiration. Evaluation of current abortion techniques is made difficult because there is a significant lag between technology and services. Asserts that early abortion should replace late abortion and contraception should replace menstrual aspiration. A major objective for all family planning programs should be the reduction of classical abortion techniques as a method of contraception.

212. <u>Planned Parenthood Response to the "Silent Scream."</u> Planned Parenthood of Seattle and Kings County, Washington, 1985. 15 min., b/w, VHS.
A number of physicians criticize the "Silent Scream" for five inaccuracies: 1) mislabeling age of the fetus in the film 2) using larger models than the age of the fetus 3) expecting viewer to understand and see sophisticated ultrasound images 4) speed of film altered 5) attributing to fetus feelings and actions which it is incapable of doing because of limited brain capacity.

213. Risk, Abraham et al.   "Second trimester abortions: review of four procedures."   New York State Journal of Medicine   75.(June 1975):1022-1027.
681 cases of second trimester abortion are reviewed.   Techniques utilized were intra-amniotic instillation of hypertonic saline, intra-amniotic PGF2alpha, extra-amniotic PGF2alpha and classic anterior hysterotomies. Efficiency of the techniques as well as the complications are compared.

214. Saltenberger, Ann.   Every Woman has a Right to Know the Dangers of Legal Abortion.   3rd ed.   Glassboro, N.J.: Air-Plus Enterprises, 1983.
A summary of the medical hazards of abortion from an anti-abortion viewpoint. Cites both reputable research articles and anti-abortion propaganda.   Should be   used with caution.

215. Silent Scream.   Donald Smith, Executive Producer. American Portrait Films, Anaheim, Ca.   1977.   30 min.; color;   VHS.
Bernard Nathanson, M.D. narrates a film from an anti-abortion point of view showing ultrasound imaging procedure on 12-week fetus and subsequent abortion using the D & C and suction technique.   Uses emotional language throughout. {See "Planned Parenthood Response to the Silent Scream" for critique and "Eclipse of Reason," the 1987 ed. of the film}.

216. Tietze, Christopher , and   Lewit, Sarah.   "Joint program for the study of abortion(JPSA): early medical complications of legal abortion." Studies in Family Planning 3.6 (1972): 97-122.
One of the most comprehensive studies of legal abortions (42,598) in the U.S.   Also evaluates early medical complications of abortion.   66 institutions reported statistics to the JPSA from July 1, 1970-June 30,1971.   Major findings were: 1) type of patient most frequently seen was young, single, white and pregnant for the first time; 2) 3 out of 4 abortions were performed on 1st trimester patients;   3) incidence of medical complications in early abortion was   1 in 20;   4) complication rates were lowest for abortions by suction, following in ascending order by classical D & E, saline, hysterotomy and hysterectomy.

217. Wentz, Anne et al.   "Techniques of pregnancy termination Pt.I."
Obstetrical and Gynecological Survey 28.(1973): 2-18;   bibl.{See Burnett,
Lonnie for Pt.II}.
Outlines techniques used for post-conception abortion and first
trimester abortion.   Surgical evacuation is presently (1973) the method
of choice for pregnancy termination of 12 weeks gestation or less.

5

Abortion Techniques (Specific)

218. <u>Abortion (First Trimester).</u>   Medfact, Inc., producer/distributor. Massillion, Ohio. 1977. 13 min.; color; VHS.
A series of still pictures and diagrams with voice-over narration answers patients' questions regarding abortions.   Covers routine tests, techniques and possible pain of a vacuum (first trimester) abortion, risks, recovery, and   contraception.

219. "Abortion without surgery?   Using prostaglandin F2alpha." <u>Time</u> 95.(February 9, 1970): 39-40.
Preliminary report on use of prostaglandin F2alpha for abortion in women pregnant from 9-22 weeks is encouraging. Researchers in Europe suggest more experience is needed with the drug, but that it appears technique could eliminate most of the risks of surgical abortion.

220. Anderson, G.G., and Steege, J.F.   "Clinical experience using intraamniotic PGF2alpha for midtrimester abortion in 600 patients." <u>Obstetrics and Gynecology</u> 46.5 (1975): 591-595; bibl.
A series of 600 patients received intraamniotic prostaglandin F2alpha to induce midtrimester abortion. 460 were complete, 140 were incomplete, and there were no abortion failures. Intraamniotic PGF2alpha is judged a safe and relatively   simple method of inducing midtrimester abortion.

221. Atienza, Milagros F. "Menstrual extraction." <u>American Journal of Obstetrics and Gynecology</u> 121.(1975): 490-495; bibl.
A clinical course of 137 consecutive menstrual extractions is described. Authors praise the use of "soft" instrumentation but caution that the

technique should be used only by trained obstetricians-gynecologists. In addition, they recommend value of simultaneous multiple pregnancy tests at different levels of sensitivity prior to menstrual extraction.

222. Barr, Maxwell M. "Mid-trimester abortion: 12-20 weeks by dilatation and evacuation method under local anesthesia." Advances in Planned Parenthood 13.(1978): 16-20; bibl.
A total of 900 patients were included in the study of the use of the D & E method for midtrimester abortion. Describes abortion techniques used and recommends the procedure for experienced surgeons within a hospital setting. The D & E method has lower mortality and failure rates, a shorter time for completion, and fewer gastrointestinal side effects. Barr feels further studies are needed on the long-term consequences of the D & E and alternative methods.

223. Bendel, Richard P. et al. "Endometrial aspiration in fertility control." American Journal of Obstetrics and Gynecology 14.4 (June 1976): 328-332; bibl.
Reports on 500 patients who received endometrial aspiration within 5-21 days following failure of expected menstruation. Histologic examination revealed that approximately one-third of the patients were not pregnant at the time of the aspiration. Serious side effects were minimal and limited to 1% infection rate.

224. Berger, G.S. et al. "Oxytocin administration, instillation-to-abortion time, and morbidity associated with saline instillation." American Journal of Obstetrics and Gynecology 121.(1975): 941-946; bibl.
A study of 4,069 women undergoing saline abortion shows that patients administered oxytocin had a shorter instillation-to-abortion time (median, 25.5 hrs) than did patients not adminstered oxytocin (median 33.3 hours). Reduction in time occurred only when oxytocin was administered within 8 hours after saline instillation. A disadvantage of the procedure is the apparent risk of clinical consumptive coagulopathy associated with aborting the fetus within 24 hours after instillation of hypertonic saline.

225. Berger, G.S. et al. "Termination of pregnancy by "super coils":
morbidity   associated with a new method of second trimester abortion."
American Journal   of Obstetrics and Gynecology 116.(1973): 297-304;
bibl.
An approximate 60% morbidity rate for a series of women who had been
aborted with the insertion of a "super coil" conflicts with earlier
literature about its safety.   Authors stress tests on new abortion
methods should be conducted in a careful scientific setting using
competent medical personnel.

226. Beric, B.   "The Karman catheter: a preliminary evaluation as an
instrument for the termination of pregnancies up to 12 weeks gestation."
American Journal of Obstetrics and Gynecology 114.(1972): 273-275;
bibl.
Concludes the catheter offers the advantage of no dilatation and
anesthesia for most early pregnancies but is not suitable for terminating
pregnancies beyond the sixth week of gestation.

227. Bongaarts, John, and Tietze, Christopher.   "Efficiency of menstrual
regulation as a method of fertility control."   Studies in Family Planning
8.(1977): 268-272;   bibl.
Using a computer simulation as an analytical tool, authors estimate the
number of menstrual regulation procedures required per 1,000 women per
year, the number required to prevent one live birth, and the percent of
procedures performed on women who are not pregnant but whose periods
are delayed.   The efficacy of menstrual regulation is also compared with
induced abortion performed later in the first trimester of pregnancy.
The number of procedures required, the costs and possible risks are all
reduced if abortion or menstrual regulation is used as a backup to
contraception.

228. Borell, U. et al.   "Successful first trimester abortion following the
use of 15 (S) 15 methyl-prostaglandin F2alpha methyl ester vaginal
suppositories." Contraception 13.(1976): 87-94.
58 women in a Swedish study had successful abortions following serial
self-adminstration of 15-me-PGF2alpha me-ester and a vacuum
aspiration.   Authors suggest in the future that this method of
self-administration may be possible   without operative interference.

229. Brenner, William E. et al.   "Menstrual regulation in the U.S.:   a preliminary report."   Fertility and Sterility 26.3 (March 1975): 289-295; bibl.
The efficacy and safety of vacuum aspiration on an outpatient basis within 14 days of a missed menstrual period was evaluated.   The failure rate was 4.2%.   Complications appeared to be less frequent and severe than complications associated with first-trimester abortions after seven weeks' gestation.

230. Brenner, William E., and Edelman, D.A.   "Dilatation and evacuation at 13 to 15 weeks' gestation versus intra-amniotic saline after 15 weeks' gestation."   Contraception 10.(1974): 171+.
To evaluate the clinical practice of deferring abortion in patients at 13-15 weeks' gestation for abortion by intra-amniotic saline at gestations of 16 weeks or over, the complication rates for 338 gravidas were compared.   In the 13-15 week period, vacuum aspiration is associated with significantly higher rates of cervical injury and the need for secondary procedures to complete the abortion when compared to D & C.   The saline method appeared to be associated with higher rates of potentially serious complications(infections, pulmonary problems) and the need for additional procedures to complete the abortion.

231. Buckle, A.E.R. et al.   "Vacuum aspiration of the uterus in therapeutic abortion."   British Medical Journal 2.(May 23, 1970): 456-457.
A study of 400 cases of therapeutic abortion by vacuum aspiration revealed few negative results.   Most patients were discharged within 24 hours of operation.   Advises against routine curettage as a conclusion to vacuum aspiration.

232. Burkman, Ronald T. et al.   "Management of midtrimester abortion failures by vaginal evacuation."   Obstetrics and Gynecology 49.(February, 1977): 233-235; bibl.
The management of 58 failed second trimester abortions by vaginal uterine evacuation is described.   The indications, techniques, and complications of this procedure are described.

233. Bygdeman, M.   et al.   "Self-administration of prostaglandin for

termination of early pregnancy." Contraception 24.1 (July, 1981): 45-52; bibl.

In a pilot study, 40 women in Sweden with a positive pregnancy test and an amenorrhea of less than 50 days and at least one previous pregnancy were selected for a legal termination of pregnancy. The patients treated themselves at home with two suppositories containing PGE2 at 6 hr. intervals. All patients but 1 (98%) aborted completely. 16 patients (40%) had no side effects, while 50% of the patients had occasional episodes of vomiting and/or diarrhea. 35% of the patients received analgesics for uterine pain. Almost all patients had a positive attitude to the treatment.

234. Bygdeman, M., and Bergstrom, Sune. "Clinical use of Prostaglandins for Pregnancy Termination." Population Reports Series G.   Washington, D.C.: George Washington University Medical Center, September, 1976. 7 p.; bibl.

Clinical studies in Sweden regarding the use of prostaglandins suggests that vaginal and oral methods of administering prostaglandins in the first trimester offer a potential for safe administration, but further development is necessary. During the second trimester, abortion induced by prostaglandin administration occurred within shorter intervals of time and showed less serious complications.

235. Cadesky, K.I. et al. "Dilation and evacuation: a preferred method of midtrimester abortion." American Journal of Obstetrics and Gynecology 139.(1981): 329; bibl.

A comparison between two groups (each 29 women), one undergoing abortion by D & E and one undergoing abortion by prostaglandin F2alpha showed the superiority of the D & E method. There was a significantly lower complication rate (6.9% versus 55%) and a shorter hospital stay of one full day in the D & E group.

236. Cates, Willard Jr. et al. "Dilatation and evacuation procedures and second-trimester abortions: the role of physician skill and hospital setting." Journal of the American Medical Association 248.#5 (August 6, 1982): 559-563;   bibl.

Authors analyzed 24,664 abortions performed during 1973-1978 at a large outpatient facility. 15% of the abortions were second-trimester procedures. D & E showed a lower rate of serious complications per 100 procedures than instillation of either prostaglandin F2alpha or hypertonic saline. Concludes that while D & E requires more operator skill than suction curettage procedures, with appropriate training gynecologists can perform the technique more safely than the alternative instillation procedures and in ambulatory surgical settings when backed up by hospital facilities.

237. Cates, Willard Jr. et al. "World Health Organization studies of prostaglandins versus saline as abortifacients: a reappraisal." Obstetrics and Gynecology 52.(1978): 493-8; bibl.
A comparison of the seven World Health Organization (WHO) Task Forces protocol on the use of prostaglandins and the study from the Joint Program for the Study of Abortion under the auspices of the Center for Disease Control (JPSA/CDC) shows that D & E is safer, more convenient and less expensive than prostaglandins for abortions after 12 weeks' gestation. For abortions of more than 17 weeks' gestation, the occurrence of live births in prostaglandin induced abortions has produced serious legal and ethical problems. Authors recommend D & E be used until the effectiveness of prostaglandin regimens is established.

238. Chez, Ronald A. "Menstrual regulation/ vacuum abortion: a valid distinction?" Contraception 9.6 (June 1974): 643-649; bibl.
Examination of records of women undergoing menstrual extraction or vacuum aspiration indicates that women in both groups are epidemiologically similar. Also, authors found surgical techniques for the procedures varied from physician to physician and therefore statistics cannot be compared.

239. Corlett, Robert C., and Ballard, Charles A. "The induction of midtrimester abortion with intra-amniotic prostaglandin F2alpha : a single dose technique." American Journal of Obstetrics and Gynecology 118.(1974): 353-357.
Prostaglandin F2alpha was administered by a single intra-amniotic instillation of 40 mg. for midtrimester abortion. Of 30 patients, 15 aborted completely, 14 incompletely, and 1 failed to abort. Authors suggest prostaglandin as an alternative to hypertonic saline for second trimester abortion.

240. "Current status of the use of prostaglandins in induced abortion (editorial)." American Journal of Public Health 63. (March 1973): 189-190;   bibl.
Prostaglandins offer no practical advantages over techniques currently used in first trimester abortions; in addition, they have high levels of incidence of side effects.   They do offer significant advantages in late abortions.

241. Davis, Geoffrey.   "Mid-trimester abortion." Lancet 2.(1972): 1026.
In a letter to the editor, describes a series of 500 abortions he performed using a D & E technique similar to Dr. Slome (see his "Termination of Pregnancy")with the exceptions that he omitted use of laminaria tents and used general anesthesia throughout the procedures. No infections or readmissions occurred as a result of this procedure.

242. Early Abortion: The Earlier the Better.   Milner-Fenwick, Inc., Timonium, Md. (OB-GYN Health Series). 9 min.; color, VHS. [n.d.]
Brief group discussion, followed by explanation of an early abortion procedure through use of cartoon drawings and patient undergoing (simulated?) abortion procedure.   Mentions complications to watch for, and birth control methods.

243. Edelman, D.A. et al.   "The effectiveness and complications of abortion by dilatation and vacuum aspiration versus dilatation and rigid metal curettage." American Journal of Obstetrics and Gynecology 119.(June 15, 1974): 473-480; bibl.
Evaluations of 4,463 patients who underwent abortion at 7-19 weeks gestation. Before 9 weeks VA appears to be safer than D & C, but after 12 weeks' gestation VA is associated with higher rates of uterine injury and excessive blood loss.   At 9-12 weeks' gestation there is little difference in the overall complication rates of the two procedures.

244. Finks, Arnold A.   "Mid-trimester abortion." Lancet 1.(February 3, 1973): 263-264.
Letter to editor tells of 2,000 midtrimester abortions using local anesthesia, dilatation, and adequate ovum forceps. Claims technique was more satisfactory than the two-stage termination with laminaria tents.

245. Fortney, Judith A. et al.   "Competing risks of unnecessary procedures and complications."   <u>Studies in Family Planning</u> 8.10 (October, 1977): 257-262;   bibl.
The menstrual regulation clinic which uses positive pregnancy tests to determine both the timing and advisability of menstrual regulation procedures can reduce both the number of unnecessary procedures and the associated complications.   The exact numbers by which these unnecessary procedures are reduced will depend on the distribution of women by number of days' delay in onset of menstruation.

246. Golditch, Ira M., and Solberg, Norman.   "Induction of midtrimester abortio with intraamniotic urea, intravenous oxytocin and laminaria." <u>Journal of Reproductive Medicine</u> 15.(1975): 225-228;   bibl.
Midtrimester abortion was accomplished in 75 patients by the intraamniotic instillation of 80 g of urea and the intravenous administration of oxytocin.   In 33 of the patients, laminaria tents were inserted into the cervix.   No severe complications occurred.   The intracervical insertion of tents of laminaria digitata has shortened the instillation-abortion interval significantly.

247. Goldsmith, Sadja, and Margolis, Alan J.   "Menstrual induction." <u>Advances in Planned Parenthood</u> 9.(1974): 7-10; bibl.
Presents experience with 200 women at the University of California, San Francisco who underwent menstrual induction.   All were within 2 weeks of a missed menses, feared pregnancy and had not had a pregnancy test. Menstrual induction was   performed under paracervical block.   Authors do not advise procedure as a simple "irreversible" pregnancy test because it does involve risk.   However, the advantage of the approach lies in the immediate relief given to an extremely anxious woman whose life circumstances may make delay especially stressful.

248. Greenhalf, J.O. et al.   "Induction of therapeutic abortion by intra-amniotic injection of urea."   <u>British Medical Journal</u> I.(1971): 28-29.
Authors report preliminary experience with a new abortion technique.   10 patients (mean gestational age 17.8 weeks, calculated from the first day of the last menstrual period) were treated with an intra-amniotic injection of urea.   The mean interval between injection and abortion was

59 hours.

249.   Grimes, David A. et al.   "Midtrimester abortion by dilatation and evacuation: a safe and practical alternative."   New England Journal of Medicine 296.20 (May 19, 1977): 1141-1145; bibl.
Compares 6213 midtrimester (after 12th week of pregnancy) abortions by D & E and 8662 abortions by intra-amniotic instillation of saline. Abortions by D & E had a lower rate for major complications, including antibiotic administration, blood transfusion, and curettage or manual evacuation of the uterus.   Although large, randomized trials are needed, this method appears safe through the 20th week of pregnancy.

250. Grimes, David A. et al.   "Midtrimester abortion by dilatation and evacuation versus intra-amniotic instillation of prostaglandin F2alpha :a randomized clinical trial ."   American Journal of Obstetrics and Gynecology 137.(August, l980): 785-790.
A randomized clinical trial with 100 subjects estimated to be l3-l8 menstrual weeks pregnant indicated that D&E abortion had significantly better compliance and less delay and was more acceptable to women than instillation of F2alpha.

251.   Grimes, David A. et al.   "Midtrimester abortion by intraamniotic prostaglandin F2alpha : safer than saline?" Obstetrics and Gynecology 49.(1977): 612-6l6; bibl.
An analysis of 1241 PGF2alpha and 10,013 saline abortions shows that abortion by saline instillation was significantly safer than PGF2alpha. Saline abortions also required treatment of complications less than PGF2alpha abortions.

252. Grimes, David A., and Cates, Willard.   "The comparative efficacy and safety of intraamniotic prostaglandin F2alpha and hypertonic saline for second trimester abortion." Journal of Reproductive Medicine 22.5 (May,1979): 248-254; bibl.
A review of 15 reports comparing hypertonic saline and prostaglandin F2alpha suggests that while PGF2 alpha induces abortion faster than saline, it is also associated with higher rates of complications such as incomplete evacuation and hemorrhage.   The reports do not substantiate

the claim that PGF2alpha is superior to saline for use in abortion.

253. Gutknect, G.D., and Southern, E.M. "Termination of human pregnancy with prostaglandin analogs." Journal of Reproductive Medicine 15.(1975): 93-96;   bibl.
Reviews use of prostaglandins as a method of pregnancy termination. The major difference among the analogs is the type and incidence of side effects.   Notes that studies are continuing to improve therapy further by investigating optimal dosage levels to lower or eliminate side-effects.

254. Hale, Ralph W. et al.   "Vaginal administration of prostaglandins to induce early abortion." Advances in the Biosciences 9.(1973): 561-565.
A small study of 20 patients whose pregnancies were terminated by the use of intravaginal prostaglandin PGF2alpha revealed mixed results. Although the administration of prostaglandin was simple, abortions were not complete in 15 patients.   Authors recommend further study of the drug and its use.

255. Hern, Warren M.   "Outpatient second-trimester D & E abortion through 24 menstrual weeks' gestation." Advances in Planned Parenthood 16.(1981): 7-13;   bibl.
Experience with 1,000 patients with gestational ages ranging from 13-26 menstrual weeks showed that abortions performed by D & E following serial laminaria treatment and urea infusion can safely be performed for advanced gestations on an outpatient basis.

256. Hodari, A.A. et al.   "Dilation and curettage for second-trimester abortions." American Journal of Obstetrics and Gynecology 127.(1977): 850.
Results of 2,500 second trimester abortions performed by D & C indicates that the procedure is safer and less traumatic than intrauterine saline or prostaglandin instillation.   Also noted was low incidence of uterine perforation;   low incidence of all-over morbidity; and short hospital stay (average of 1.1 days per patient).

257. Hodgson, Jane E. "Menstrual extraction." JAMA 228.7 (May 13,

1974):   849-850;   bibl.
Claims that the actual techniques for menstrual extraction are the same
as those used in early abortion and that the profession should
acknowledge the technique as another form of "abortion" rather than
calling it something else.   Urges against use of non-physicians to
perform technique and cautions necessity for pregnancy testing before
procedure to avoid unnecessary extractions.

258. Hodgson, Jane E.   "Reassessment of menstrual regulation."   Studies
in   Family Planning 8.(1977): 263-267;   bibl.
Author reports changes in thinking regarding menstrual regulation since
the first international conference on menstrual regulation held in
Honolulu, December, 1973.   Because of the risks involved, menstrual
regulation without confirmation of pregnancy is not advised where
reliable testing is available.   A better decision is to wait until
conventional pregnancy tests are reliable, at six weeks since last
menstrual period.

259. Holtrop, Hugh R., and Waite, Ronald S.   Uterine Aspiration Techniques
in   Family Planning.   Boston, Mass.: The Pathfinder Fund, 1976.   67 p.;
bibl.
Surveys history of uterine aspiration, followed by a review of female
reproductive anatomy and the physiology of early pregnancy.   The new
equipment systems for uterine aspiration and minimum standards for
clinic personnel and facilities are described.   Cites results of recent
clinical studies.

260. Irani, Katy R. et al.   "Menstrual induction: its place in clinical
practice."   Obstetrics and Gynecology 46.5 (November, 1975): 596-598;
bibl.
From June, 1973-October 1974 221 patients underwent menstrual
induction in a   private office setting.   Pregnancy tests were given prior
to the procedure, which took place 7-21 days after expected menstrual
period.   98.2% of the patients proved pregnant on histologic examination
of the removed tissue.   The complication rates were acceptably low.

261. Karim, S.M.M., and   Filshie, G.M.   "Therapeutic abortion using

prostaglandin F2alpha." Lancet i.7639 (January 24, 1970): 157-159; bibl.
15 patients were treated with intravenous infusions of prostaglandin F2alpha. The gestational age varied between 9 and 22 weeks. Abortion was successful in 14 cases and complete in 13. Diarrhea and vomiting were the only side-effects noted. Authors recommend that a larger clinical trial be performed.

262. Karman, Harvey , and Potts. Malcolm. "Very early abortion using syringe as vacuum source." Lancet i.(May 13, 1972): 1051-1052.
Vacuum aspiration is becoming the preferred method for terminating pregnancy during the first 12 weeks of gestation (up to 7 weeks from the last menstrual period). The simplest apparatus is a 50 ml. syringe directly connected to a 5 or 6 mm. external diameter Karman cannula. Care must be taken to limit the procedure to where the uterus is only slightly enlarged and to women who have no complicating pelvic disease or abnormalities.

263. Keirse, Marc J.N.C. et al. Second Trimester Pregnancy Termination. Boerhaave series for postgraduate medical education 22. The Hague: Leiden University Press, 1982. 210 p.; bibl.
Discusses suitable methods of termination of pregnancy in the second trimester, including handling of complications, potential risks and long-term effects. Consideration is given to the demographic and legal effects of termination of pregnancy in the second trimester, as well as factors responsible for delay in securing abortion and provision of postabortion contraception.

264. Kerenyi, Thomas D. et al. "Flve thousand consecutive saline inductions." American Journal of Obstetrics and Gynecology 116.(1973): 593-600; bibl.
5,000 consecutive saline inductions were performed without maternal death. The serious complications associated with this technique in the literature, i.e., convulsions, coma, and cerebral damage, were not encountered. This is attributed to the use of the slow drip infusion method and strict adherence to established guidelines. Complications related to labor and delivery are tabulated and discussed.

265. Kessel, Elton et al.   "Menstrual regulation in family planning."
American Journal of Public Health 65.7 (July 1975): 731-734; bibl.
Evaluates menstrual regulation as safe, effective and economic.   Its
increased safety as compared with first trimester abortion makes it a
better medical practice for the time of up to 14 days missed menstrual
period.   Acceptance of the practice will depend on availability,
information about the service and ability of women to use the service
without delay.

266. Lauersen, Niels H.   "Midtrimester abortion induced with a single
intra-amniotic instillation of prostaglandin F2alpha." American Journal
of Obstetrics and Gynecology 118.(1974): 210-217; bibl.
Midtrimester abortion was successfully induced in 20 patients with a
single instillation of 40 mg. of prostaglandin F2alpha administered over
a 10 minute period.   The mean abortion time was 16.24 hours which
compares favorably with the results of saline-induced abortions.   17
patients aborted completely and 3 incompletely and side-effects
appeared less frequently than when midtrimester abortion was
performed with serial PGF2alpha instillations.

267. Laufe, Leonard E. , and Kreutner, A. Karen. "Vaginal hysterectomy: a
modality for therapeutic abortion and sterilization."   American Journal
of Obstetrics and Gynecology 3.(1971): 1096-1099.
Vaginal hysterectomy is an effective and safe procedure for the patient
requiring therapeutic abortion and sterilization.   A series of 71
consecutive patients underwent this procedure at the Western
Pennsylvania Hospital from 1961-1970.   The most frequent complication
was urinary infection.

268. Lewis, Stella C. et al.   "Outpatient termination of pregnancy."
British Medical Journal 4.(1971): 606-610; bibl.
Termination of pregnancies ranging from 6-10 weeks gestation is
described for 127 women who were at Kings College Hospital in London
as outpatients.   The technique used was a Karman catheter.   The early
high incidence of postoperative complications altered the practice from
catheter alone to curetting with a small Friedman curette after the use
of the Karman catheter.   In addition, local anesthetic was later employed
after an initial trial of no anesthesia.   Both paracervical and

intracervical block eliminated the pain of inserting the catheter, while some local uterine discomfort remained while suction was applied.

269.   Lewit, Sarah.   "D & E midtrimester abortion: a medical innovation." Women and Health 7.1 (Spring 1982) 49-55; bibl.
Discusses the changes in pregnancy termination procedures between 1973-1982.   About 85% of all early midtrimester abortions and about 25% of abortions at 16 weeks' gestation were done by D & E in 1978. Very few medical schools include D & E procedures in their residency training program.

270. Lewit, Sarah . "Sterilization associated with induced abortion: JPSA findings." Family Planning Perspectives 5.3 (Summer, 1973): 177-182; bibl.
Results from the Joint Program for the Study of Abortion (JPSA) indicate that 3.7% of the women who had abortions also underwent sterilization. The proportions sterilized increased sharply with the woman's age and parity.   Women on nonprivate service and nonwhite women were sterilized more frequently at younger ages and lower parities than were women on private service and white women.

271. Loung, K.C. et al. "Results in 1,000 cases of therapeutic abortion managed by vacuum aspiration." British Medical Journal 4.(November 20, 1971): 477-479.
Study of 1,000 cases managed by vacuum aspiration confirms the value and safety of the technique.   Uterine perforation was encountered in 5 patients, and hemorrhage in excess of 500 ml. occurred in 6% of the patients.

272. Martin, J.N. et al.   "Early second trimester abortion by the extraamniotic instillation of Rivanol solution and a single PGF2alpha dose." Contraception 11.(1975): 523-531.
The induction of early second trimester abortion by extra-amniotic instillation of a single dose of prostaglandin(PGF2alpha) in a solution of 0.1% Rivanol seems to be a simple procedure.   The pilot study of 26 patients indicates that the procedure eliminates the necessity for repeat administrations of a primary prostaglandin compound and has acceptable

side-effects.

273. Mattingly, Richard F. "The paramedic abortionist." Obstetrics and Gynecology 41.(June 1973): 929-930.
Disputes Karman's claim (see Karman citations) that the "super coil" abortion method is suitable for use by paramedic personnel. States that the method carries higher major and total complication rates than the method of saline-amniotic fluid exchange.

274. Miller, Eva et al. "Early vacuum aspiration: minimizing procedures to nonpregnant women." Family Planning Perspectives 8.1 (1976): 33-38; bibl.
Using data collected by the International Fertility Research Program, the authors analyze results from 8,000 vacuum aspirations in order to present a decision-making model for future patients requesting vacuum aspiration after delayed menses of 0-14 days. The authors recommend an aspiration procedure for all patients who have a positive pregnancy test. In addition, they recommend delaying the procedure for one week for those patients whose tests are indefinite or negative. This delay can eliminate three-fifths of unnecessary procedures.

275. Moghadam, S.S. et al. "A comparison of metal and plastic cannulae for performing vacuum aspiration during the first trimester of pregnancy." The Journal of Reproductive Medicine 17.(1976): 181-187; bibl.
A comparative study to determine the efficacy of a metal or flexible plastic 8mm cannula for induced abortion at 6-10 weeks gestation showed no significant differences in complication rates between the two groups of subjects. Physicians' choice may be based on such factors as experience, personal preference, cost and availability.

276. Nathanson, Bernard M. "Ambulatory abortion, experience with 26,000 cases." New England Journal of Medicine 286.(1972): 403-407; bibl.
Presents data from the Center for Reproductive and Sexual Health for July 1,1970-August 1,1971. Abortions were performed by the vacuum-aspiration technique under paracervical-block anesthesia. No

deaths resulting from the technique are reported.   Preabortion counseling was successful in lessening preabortion stress.

277. Nathanson, Bernard N.   "Drugs for the production of abortion: a review."   Obstetrical and Gynecological Survey 25.(1970): 727-731; bibl. Reviews literature on abortifacient drugs and concludes that there is no safe, reliable drug at present (1970) which will cause termination of pregnancy.

278. Newman, Lucille, and Murphy, Maureen.   "Menstrual induction: II. Psychosocial aspects."   Advances in Planned Parenthood 9.(1974): 11-14; bibl.
Authors reviewed the counseling aspect on menstrual induction patients (see Goldsmith, Sadja for medical aspects).   113 women were interviewed before the induction and given a "pain card" to fill out after the induction which compared a normal menstrual period with a menstrual induction experience.   The majority of respondents described any pain they felt during the menstrual induction as similar to or more intense than during a regular period and not lasting as long. Concedes importance of procedure for the relief it gives extremely anxious patients, and suggests counseling can be aimed towards the single, non-sexually active patient.

279. Novak, F., and Andolsek, L., eds. Comparison of the Medical Effects of Induced Abortion by Two Methods: Curettage and Vacuum Aspiration. Bethesda, Md.: National Institutes of Health, Center for Population Research, 1974. 57 p.
A comparison study of the medical effects of induced abortion by curettage (D & C) and vacuum aspiration (VA) was carried out on a group of 4733 women in Yugoslavia.   Major recommendations as a result of the study are: 1) VA is better than D & C because it has a lower perforation rate, induces less blood loss and involves less subsequent infections which require hospitalization 2) VA should be performed within the first 10 weeks of pregnancy 3) objective evaluations of complications must be obtained from medical records rather than from the patients themselves.

280. Penfield, A. J.   "Abortion under paracervical block."   New York State

Journal of Medicine 71.(1972): 1185-1189.
The author performed more than 600 first trimester abortions by dilitation and suction followed by instrumental curettage under paracervical block.   He analyzes results from a series of 291 first trimester abortions, 187 in the Planned Parenthood Center and 104 in the physician's office.   There were 5 complications in the series.   He concludes this method is safe and effective for an outpatient facility.

281. Roberts, G. et al.   "Therapeutic abortion by intra-amniotic injection of prostaglandins." British Medical Journal 4.(October 7, 1972): 12-14.
Intra-amniotic injections of either prostaglandin F2alpha or prostaglandin E2 were used to induced therapeutic abortion in 27 patients.   Termination of pregnancy was successful in 11 out of 13 when prostaglandin E2 alone was used, but in only 6 out of 14 when prostaglandin F2alpha was used.   The technique was judged safe when E2 was used, but the authors propose to abandon the use of F2alpha because of its disappointing results in the trial. The best method of administering prostaglandins also remains uncertain.

282. Rooks, Judith Bourne , and Cates, Willard Jr.   "Emotional impact of D & E versus instillation."   Family Planning Perspectives 9.(Nov/Dec. l973):   276-277.
Considers D & E procedure as less expensive, less painful, and less emotionally traumatic for the patient than instillation.

283. Schulman, Harold et al.   "Outpatient saline abortion."   Obstetrics & Gynecology 37.4 (April 1971): 521-526; bibl.
A clinical study of 323 women who underwent saline abortion with the option of aborting at home demonstrated that morbidity was equal to or less than that reported for abortions administered on an inpatient basis. Patients did not appear to experience psychological distress from aborting at home rather than in a hospital.

284. Scotti, Richard J., and Karman, Harvey L.   "Menstrual regulation and early pregnancy termination performed by paraprofessionals under medical supervision." Contraception 14.4 (1976): 367-374; bibl.
774 patients whose gestational size was 10 weeks or less were aspi-

rated with a Karman cannulae attached to a modified 50cc vacuum syringe. The clinic used a physician and 8 women paramedics under medical supervision to perform the procedures, which had a 1.3% complication rate. Concludes menstrual regulation up to 10 weeks gestation can be performed by trained paramedical personnel in a clinical setting under medical supervision.

285. Slome, John. "Termination of pregnancy." Lancet 2.(1972): 881-882.
A short letter to the editor describes a series of 50 patients (16-20 weeks pregnant) who underwent abortion by the D & E method using laminaria tents for the dilatation. States that this method is preferable to intrauterine infusion of prostaglandins.

286. Sood, S.V. "Termination of pregnancy by the interuterine insertion of Utus paste." British Medical Journal ii.(1971): 315-317; bibl.
Utus paste was used to induce abortion in 83 women. Pain was a prominent symptom in many cases. Complications included 3 cases of septicaemia and one death. Author concludes the method is too dangerous to justify its future use.

287. Southern, E.M., and Gutknecht, G.D. "The use of prostaglandins for the therapeutic termination of pregnancy." Journal of Reproductive Medicine 13.(1974): 63-66; bibl.
Reviews methods of administration and dosage levels for prostaglandins and lists complications for each method. Concludes that prostaglandins "have appeared as rather profound newcomers in the total realm of population control."

288. Stim, Edward M. "Saline abortion." Obstetrics and Gynecology 40.2 (1972): 247-251; bibl.
Among 612 intraamniotic saline injections given at a New York hospital, 97.4% induced successful abortions. The problems encountered included a high incidence of retained placenta and postabortion hemorrhage.

289. Stroh, George, and Hinman, Alan R. "Reported live births following

induced abortion: two and one-half years' experience in Upstate New York." <u>American Journal of Obstetrics and Gynecology</u> 126.(1976): 83-90; bibl.
38 live births following induced abortion were recorded in Upstate New York between July 1970-December 1972. 26 followed saline-induced abortions. Underestimate of gestation and inadequate saline-amniotic procedures seemed to account for the births.

290. Stubblefield, Phillip G. et al. "Randomized study of 12mm and 15.9mm canullas in midtrimester abortion by laminaria and vacuum curettage." <u>Fertility and Sterility</u> 29.(May, 1973): 512-517; bibl.
Study of the efficacy of the large-bore vacuum cannula system for midtrimester abortion (13-16 weeks gestation) proved the procedure safe and more acceptable to physicians than amnioinfusion of hypertonic saline or prostaglandin F2alpha.

291. Van den Vlugt, Theresa, and Piotrow, P.T. "Menstrual Regulation: What is it?" <u>Population Reports</u>. 9-21; Series F. 9-21; bibl. George Washington University Medical Center: Dept. of Medical and Public Affairs, April,1973.
Reviews techniques and equipment used in menstrual regulation. Advantages to the procedure are its safety, simplicity, low-cost and few complications. Two controversies are: should the procedure be performed when a pregnancy is probable though not positively established, and is there a danger that menstrual regulation will be used as a substitute for contraception?

292. Van den Vlugt, Theresa, and Piotrow, P.T. "Menstrual Regulation Update." <u>Population Reports.</u> Series F. 49-64; bibl. George Washington University Medical Center: Dept. of Medical and Public Affairs, May, 1974.
Summary of a three-day conference on menstrual regulation held on December 17-19, 1973 in Honolulu, Hawaii. Highlight of the conference was the statistical analysis of low rates of complications and failures of the procedure. Of 3,490 women for whom detailed data were available in December,1973, 74 (or 2.12 per 100 women) experienced complications. This compares favorably with a previous (April 1973) complication rate of 4.7 per 100 women based on similar complications in 74 out of 1544 cases. Also discusses therapeutic uses for menstrual

regulation. Participants recommend that menstrual regulation should be fully integrated not only with maternal health and family planning programs but with general health services.

293. Van den Vlugt, Theresa, and Piotrow, P.T. "Uterine Aspiration Techniques." Population Reports ;Series F. 25-48; bibl. Washington, D.C.: George Washington University Medical Center, June, 1973.
Reviews uterine aspiration techniques, including history, pre and post operative procedures, complications, mortality and equipment. Charts of selected studies on uterine aspiration compare and contrast clinical results.

294. WHO Task Force on the Use of Prostaglandins for the Regulation of Fertility. "Comparison of intraamniotic prostaglandin F2alpha and hypertonic saline for induction of second-trimester abortion." British Medical Journal 1.(June 5, 1976): 1373-1376; bibl.
In an international multicenter randomized study, the efficacy and safety of intraamniotic prostaglandin and hypertonic saline were compared. The main advantage of PGF2alpha was its significantly higher success rates in the first 48 hours. Side effects were within acceptable limits.

295. Williford, J.F., and Wheeler, R.G. "Advances in non-electrical vacuum equipment for uterine aspiration." Advances in Planned Parenthood 9.(1975): 74-82; bibl.
New techniques of nonelectrical uterine aspiration in the form of the modified Karman syringe, the automatic negative pressure bottle and the hand-pumped aspirator have been advantageous from the standpoint of lowering equipment costs and reducing the complexity of aspiration systems.

296. Wong, Ting-Chao, and Schulman, Harold. "Endometrial aspiration as a means of early abortion." Obstetrics and Gynecology 44.6 (December 1974): 845-852; bibl.
A study of endometrial aspiration as a means of early abortion showed a complication rate of 4.2%, none a major type. Although approximately 15% of the patients were not pregnant, authors believe the safety and simplicity of the procedure justifies its use.

6

Counseling

297. Addelson, Frances. "Induced abortion: source of guilt or growth?"
American Journal of Orthopsychiatry 43.5 (October 1973): 815-823.
Social work service with pregnancy clinic patients suggests the need for
continued involvement in counseling. The goal of psychological recovery
needs to be an integral part of the abortion experience.

298. Anwyl, J.H.   "The role of private counseling for problem
pregnancies." Clinical Obstetrics and Gynecology 14.(December 1971):
1225-1229;   bibl.
Explores counseling procedures for abortion clinics, stating that private
counseling can help the patient consider how maximum freedom and
responsibility are to be achieved.   Abortion counseling should be
followed up with contraceptive counseling.

299. Asher, John D. "Abortion counseling."   American Journal of Public
Health 62.5 (May 1972): 686-688; bibl.
Aims of abortion counseling are to help the woman make her decision,
implement it, and assist her in controlling her future fertility.   Training
programs for counselors must include work in the areas of human
sexuality and psychology and observation and practice sessions with
trainees.

300. Bauer, Herbert. "Abortion counseling: before, after and again."
Medical Insight 6.(January 1974): 8-11.
Stressses need to have continuum of abortion services from diagnosis to
post-abortion counseling.   What matters most is the counselor's attitude
towards abortion and towards the patient.

301. Bernstein, Norman R. , and   Tinkham, Caroline B.   "Group therapy following abortion."   Journal of Nervous and Mental Disease 152.5 (May, 1971): 303-314;   bibl.
Authors worked with a group of 20 women who had received abortions. They met once a week for 13 weeks.   One mixed group of married and unmarried women was able to discuss their feelings about abortion and to support each other, share ideas and help resolve conflicts.   In contrast, another group of single girls seemed unable to develop mutual relationships or to sustain an effective therapy group.   For both groups it seemed clear that the abortions did not have a   deleterious effect on the women.

302. Bracken, Michael B. et al.   "Abortion counseling: an experimental study of three techniques."   American Journal of Obstetrics and Gynecology 117.(1973): 10-19; bibl.
489 abortion patients were randomly assigned to three different counseling procedures (group orientation, group process, and individual). Data collected were: circumstances surrounding the pregnancy; reaction to counseling session; response to abortion.   Most women preferred individual counseling.   Younger women responded to the abortion more favorably after either type of group counseling.

303. Brashear, Diane B.   "Abortion counseling."   Family Coordinator 22.4 (October, 1973): 429-435;   bibl.
Reviews recent literature on abortion counseling and indicates major issues in the field.   Includes discussion on psychological cost, decision-making process, client expectations and referral role of counselor.

304. Buckles, Nancy B.   "Abortion: a technique for working through grief." Journal of the American College Health Association 30.4 (February 1982): 181-182;   bibl.
Suggests gestalt technique for dealing with loss of fetus by having abortion patient express regrets, resentments and appreciations while saying goodbye.   In addition, second part of the process is the establishment of positive remembrance of the meaning of the fetus to the woman.

305. Burnell, George M. et al. "Post-abortion group therapy." American Journal of Psychiatry 129.(August, 1972): 220-223; bibl.
250 women who had had therapeutic abortions attended group therapy programs led by a psychiatrist and gynecologist team. The program was beneficial, helping patients to cope with guilt feelings and to clear areas of misinformation about sexual function and contraception. The program also tended to help change staff attitudes in a positive way.

306. Carmen, Arlene , and Moody, Howard. Abortion Counseling and Social Change: From Illegal Act to Medical Practice. Valley Forge: Judson Press, 1973. 122 p.
A fascinating history of the organization, Clergy Consultation Service on Abortion (CCS) which was one of the first social service agencies to help women obtain abortions.   Discusses problems encountered and the opposition of physicians, law enforcement agencies and the Catholic Church.   Also covers implementation of the new pro-abortion laws and how consultation services were set up.

307. Columbia University School of Social Work. Counseling in Abortion Services.   New York: Columbia University, 1973. 61 p.
Proceedings from a conference on counseling in the area of abortion services cover nurse, physician and social work counseling, and future needs.   Also contains observation notes on the current state of abortion counseling.

308. Cotroneo, Margaret, and Krasner, Barbara R. "A study of abortion and problems in decision-making." Journal of Marriage and Family Counseling 3.1 (January 1977): 69-76; bibl.
Clinical observations of cases of abortion reveal that pregnancy counselors tend to place a high value on a woman's individual needs. Authors recommend more attention be paid to the woman's relationships with her partner and relatives in family counseling sessions.

309. Dauber, Bonnie et al. "Abortion counseling and behavioral change." Family Planning Perspectives 4.2 (April, 1972): 23-27; bibl.
At San Francisco General Hospital, two groups of women (counseled and non-counseled) were compared to determine the results after their

abortions. Of 99 counseled women, 94 returned for a post-abortion checkup versus 60 of 99 non-counseled women. Comments were made by a number of women that the counseling provided a measure of support and helped eliminate their sense of isolation.

310. Dunlop, Joyce L. "Counselling of patients requesting an abortion." The Practitioner 220.(1978): 847-852.
Ambivalence is the most important single factor that a counsellor should be looking for in a pregnant woman who has come for help. Abortion should also be considered in schizophrenia and manic-depressive psychoses. Good counselling does not end with the decision to terminate the pregnancy but should continue before, during,and after the pregnancy.

311. Gedan, Sharon. "Abortion counseling with adolescents." American Journal of Nursing 74.10 (October 1974): 1856-1858; bibl.
A particular problem associated with counseling of adolescent abortion patients is that the women can become involved in destructive game playing with their parents. Notes importance of counseling family and partners and stresses need for contraceptive counseling.

312. Gibb, Gerald D., and Millard, Richard J. "Divergent perspectives in abortion counseling." Psychological Reports 50.3, pt. 1 (June, 1982): 819-822; bibl.
Tests given to abortion clients (and a control group), contrary to expectations, indicate that clients viewed themselves as internally controlled. Counseling directed towards helping the client have more personal control would not be useful under these circumstances.

313. Gill, Robin. "Variables in abortion counselling." British Journal of Guidance and Counselling 3.1 (January 1975): 56-65; bibl.
Examines five variables involved in abortion counseling: 1-2) religio-ethical beliefs of the counselor and counselee 3) the status of abortion laws 4) available abortion techniques 5) counselor's assumptions about the sequelae of abortion. Presents personal assessment of relative importance of the variables.

314. Gordon, Robert H.   "Efficacy of a group crisis-counseling program for men who accompany women seeking abortions." American Journal of Community Psychology 6.3 (June 1978): 239-246; bibl.
Groups of males who accompanied partners to an abortion clinic were counseled or not counseled.   On tests given on arrival and two hours later, anxiety decreased and attitudes were more positive for men in the group which received crisis counseling.

315. Hare, M.J., and Heywood, Jane. "Counselling needs of women seeking abortions." Journal of Biosocial Science 13.3 (July 1981): 269-273; bibl.
Findings in a study of 162 women requesting abortion were that over half the women needed to talk over or clarify the options in their case or to receive help or information.   In addition, some needed a helper to whom they could come back and who would support them.

316. Joffe, Carole.   "What abortion counselors want from their clients." Social Problems 26.1 (October 1978): 112-121; bibl.
After observing interactions between abortion counselors and patients, author concludes ideal client is one who does not make demands on counselors, is "sober" in behavior, and is not a repeat aborter.   Author states abortion work "may represent a class of occupational activity that will always be carried out with some ambivalence."

317. Joy, Stephany S.   "Abortion: an issue to grieve?"   Journal of Counseling and Development 63.(February 1985): 375-376.
Author found that women respond favorably to counseling using a grief format--the processing of the loss of the fetus as an unresolved grief issue.   Cautions that more data needs to be compiled with respect to long-term emotional effects.

318. Kahn-Edrington, Marla.   "Abortion counseling."   Counseling Psychologist 8.1 (1979): 37-38.
The role of the abortion counselor is to mobilize each woman's coping skills and facilitate movement toward a final, fully integrated decision. Outlines recommended principles for counselors.

319. Keller, Christa, and   Copeland, Pamela.   "Counseling the abortion patient is more than talk."   American Journal of Nursing   72.(January, 1972): 102-106; bibl.
Authors state that the concerned and sympathetic treatment of the abortion patient needs to start when the patient enters the clinic.   Staff must be hired who will be able to be supportive of the patient. Discussions about the abortion experience need to be followed up with counseling on contraception.

320. Kummer, Jerome M.   "Counseling women who are considering abortion."   Journal of Pastoral Care   25.4 (December 1971): 233-240; bibl.
Reviews historical background and changes in abortion laws which have led to a new climate for abortion counselors.   Counselors can best help women by hearing them out and permitting them to arrive at conclusions validated by having had the experience of talking with a trusted counselor.   Also stresses importance of conception control.

321. Lodl, Karen M. et al.   "Women's responses to abortion: implications for post-abortion support groups."   Journal of Social Work and Human Sexuality 3.2-3 (Winter-Spring 1984/85): 119-132; bibl. Special Issue: Feminist perspectives on social work and human sexuality.
A review of the literature on the psychological effects of abortion and implications for post-abortion counseling shows that while abortion is essentially a positive procedure it can also be stressful and emotionally difficult for some.   Counseling literature focuses on two factors: alleviation of symptoms of grief, depression, anger and guilt and bringing the abortion experience to a positive closure.   Suggests model for post-abortion support group.

322. Lubman, Alison J.   Assessment of an Intervention Program for Partners of Abortion Patients.   Boulder: University of Colorado, 1981. 212 p.
One group of men at an abortion clinic who received intervention (N=33) and a control group (N=31) who did not were compared as to various aspects of sexual and contraceptive behavior and the abortion experience. Men who received the intervention were less anxious at the time of abortion and somewhat more supportive of their partners.   However,

their attitudes towards contraception and responsibility toward contraceptive use did not change.

323. Margolis, Alan J.   "Some thoughts on medical evaluation and counseling of applicants for abortion."   Clinical Obstetrics and Gynecology 14.(Dec. 1971): 1255-1257; bibl.
Medical interview of applicants for abortion should include physical examination and laboratory tests, and counseling should include contraceptive counseling and postabortion counseling.

324. Marmer, Stephen S. et al.   "Is psychiatric consultation in abortion obsolete?" International Journal of Psychiatry in Medicine 5.3 (Summer 1974): 201-209; bibl.
Although the 1973 Supreme Court decision has eliminated the need for "routine" psychiatric evaluations, there are indications for psychiatric involvement in post-abortion counseling.   Indicative factors include ambivalence, self-destructive use of sexuality, incompetence, and history of prior psychiatric illness or suicidal behavior.

325. Naugle, Ethel. "Counseling abortion patients." Nursing 3.(February 1973): 37-38.
Outlines counseling philosophy, purposes and methods.   Goals of counseling are to provide a warm, supportive atmosphere, instructions and guidelines regarding the abortion procedure, and contraceptive advice.

326. Ness, Mary. "An appraisal of abortion counselling." British Journal of Guidance and Counselling 4.1 (January 1976): 79-87; bibl.
Describes 306 cases seen in a pregnancy advisory service, discussing aims of the service, the counseling process, problems, aftercare, medical counseling and recommendations for the future.

327. Planned Parenthood Federation of America. A Consumer's Alert to Deception, Harassment and Medical Malpractice. New York: Planned Parenthood, 1987. flyer.
Discusses how to recognize anti-abortion counseling centers and how to

locate professional pregnancy counseling centers.

328. Reichelt, Paul A., and Werley, Harriet H.   "Contraception, abortion and venereal disease: teenagers' knowledge and the effect of education." Family   Planning Perspectives 7.2 (1975): 83-88.
Studies of teenagers at a family planning clinic indicated that while most are either misinformed or uninformed about the various methods of contraception, they are well-informed about abortion and venereal diseases.   Testing after a single, informal rap session improved knowledge substantially in most areas.

329. Sanders, Raymond S. et al.   "Counseling for elective abortion." Journal of American College Health Association   21.(June 1973): 446-450;   bibl.
In order to investigate the effectiveness of a counseling and referral service at a university health clinic, questionnaires filled out by 48 women who had   undergone elective abortion were analyzed. All of the women felt the decision was appropriate, 64% without question and 36% with minor reservations.

330. Smith, Elizabeth M.   "Counseling for women who seek abortion." Social Work 17.2 (March 1972): 62-68.
46 women seeking abortion were counseled. Of these, 40 obtained abortions and were counseled again. Results were positive one week after abortion.   19 of the women were again questioned approximately one year after the abortion, with the majority of women experiencing no major emotional problems. Stresses importance of counseling for women in crisis situation.

331. Thompson, Linda V., and Robinson, Sharon E.   "Differences in self-concept and locus of control among women who seek abortions." American Mental Health   Counselors Association Journal 8.1 (January 1986): 4-11.
A study of self-concept and locus of control in three groups of women (one group seeking abortion, one group seeking contraception, and one group seeking repeat abortion) showed no significant differences in self-concept among the three groups. There were also no significant

differences in internal control, control by powerful others, and chance control.   Suggests appropriate counseling technique.

332. Ullmann, Alice.   "Social work service to abortion patients."   Social Casework 53.(October 1972): 481-487;   bibl.
Group counseling sessions were held for abortion patients in a New York hospital.   The majority of the patients were ambivalent and feelings of isolation were also apparent.   Areas requiring further study were the attitude of the professional personnel toward abortion, and the nature of emotional conflicts in patients undergoing abortion.

333. Wickwire, Karen S.   The use of a behavioral intervention in the preparation of patients for the surgical procedure involved in pregnancy termination.   University of Southern Mississippi, 1986.   104 p.
Relaxation instructions were administered to a group of 15 women out of 30 in their pre-abortion counseling sessions.   Results of the self-report, physiological, and behavioral measures of anxiety tests indicated no significant differences between the relaxation and non-relaxation groups on any of the measures.

334. Wilson, Robert R.   Problem Pregnancy and Abortion Counseling. Saluda, N.C.: Family Life Pubs., Inc., 1973. 120 p.;   bibl.
Contains essays on general counseling, principles for problem pregnancies, alternatives in continuing the pregnancy, abortion counseling, medical aspects of abortion, and contraception and reproductive education.   Appendix has resource list of organizations involved in problem pregnancy or contraceptive matters.

335. Young, Alma T. et al.   "Women who seek abortions: a study."   Social Work 18.3 (May 1973): 60-65.
A study of women at Mt. Sinai Medical Center was undertaken to determine which patients needed intensive counseling.   Two-thirds of the patients were judged to be distressed: most of the patients under 17 and three-fourths of the women 35 or older.   Patients who gave social or medical reasons for wanting an abortion were less distressed than those who gave emotional reasons.

7

Morbidity and Mortality

336. Cates, Willard Jr. et al. "Abortion deaths associated with the use of PGF2alpha." American Journal of Obstetrics and Gynecology 127.3 (1977): 219-222; bibl.
Six abortion-related deaths associated with the use of prostaglandin F2alpha were reported by the Center for Disease Control between 1972-1975. Four patients had pre-existing conditions that increased their risks and contributed to their deaths. The death-to-case ratio is approximately 10.5 per 100,000 abortions, lower than the saline ratio, but the relative safety of intra-amniotic F2alpha still remains to be established.

337. Cates, Willard Jr. "Abortion myths and realities: who is misleading whom?" American Journal of Obstetrics and Gynecology 142.8 (April 15, 1982): 954-956; bibl.
Cates points out several errors in another doctor's claim that liberal abortion laws in the United States caused more deaths among women of childbearing age than they prevented. He goes on to state that the decline of abortion mortality continued through 1976, implying that legal abortions were substituted for illegal abortions.

338. Cates, Willard Jr. , and Grimes, David A. "Deaths from second trimester abortion by dilatation and evacuation: causes, prevention, facilities." Obstetrics and Gynecology 58.4 (October, 1981): 401-408; bibl.
Reviews reported deaths from D & E in the United States between January 1, 1972 and December 31, 1978. The predominant causes of death were infection and hemorrhage. Comparative mortality data suggests abortion by D & E at 13 weeks' gestation or later is more

dangerous than suction curettage performed earlier in gestation, but safer than instillation techniques performed later.   The advantage of D & E occurs largely in the 13-15 week gestation interval.

339. Cates, Willard Jr. et al.   "The effect of delay and choice of method on the risk of abortion morbidity."   Family Planning Perspectives 9.(1977): 266-273;   bibl.
Discusses data from the Joint Program for the Study of Abortion/Center for Disease Control (JPSA/CDC) on effects of delay and method of choice on the risk of abortion morbidity.   The report on 74,254 terminations reveals that any delay increases the risk of complications and the risk appears to increase continuously and linearly as the length of the gestation increases.   D & E was more than 160 percent safer than the PGF2alpha instillation.   Concludes that acceptance of the relative safety of midtrimester D & E will reduce complications from abortions.

340. Cates, Willard Jr. et al.   "Effect of liberalized abortion on maternal mortality rates."   American Journal of Obstetrics and Gynecology 130.(1978): 372-374; bibl.
Disputes Drs. Cavanagh and Dr. Hilgers' contention that liberalized abortion laws have caused more deaths of women of childbearing ages than they have prevented.   Finds fault with Hilger for extrapolation of regression, use of noncomparable data and selection of inappropriate time intervals.   Concludes that the decline in abortion deaths increased from 11.87% (1961-1968) to 20.8%   (1968-1973).

341. Cates, Willard Jr. et al.   "Legalized abortion: effect on national trends of maternal and abortion-related mortality ratios (1940 through 1976)."   American Journal of Obstetrics and Gynecology 132.(1978): 211-214; bibl.
The maternal mortality rate, excluding abortion, has continually declined from 1940-1976 at an average annual rate of 13% before 1956 and 5% thereafter.   The abortion mortality rate ratio passed through three major phases between 1940-1976.   In the first phase (1940-1950), there was a steady decline at an average annual rate of 18%.   In the second phase (1951-1965) the abortion mortality ratio leveled off at an average annual rate of decrease of 1.7%.   Thereafter, the abortion mortality ratio decreased at an average annual rate of 11% (1966-1970) and accelerated

to 25% (1970-1976). The authors consider the increased availability of legal abortions and introduction of more effective contraception as the two most likely reasons for the accelerated decline in abortion-related deaths.

342. Cates, Willard Jr. et al. "Mortality from abortion and childbirth: are the statistics biased?" Journal of the American Medical Association 248.#2 (July 9, 1982): 192-196; bibl.
Evaluates claim of critics that biases in crude data favor the safety of abortion. Authors reviewed the sources of mortality data and examined the completeness of abortion mortality statistics, childbirth mortality statistics, and the accuracy of the denominators for both these events. Abortion deaths appear to be more completely ascertained than childbirth deaths and use of a different denominator has relatively little impact on the comparison. Concludes that crude data are biased in a direction that overestimates abortion risks relative to the risks of childbearing.

343. Cates, Willard Jr., and Jordaan, Harold V. "Sudden collapse and death of women obtaining abortions induced with prostaglandin F2alpha." American Journal of Obstetrics and Gynecology 133.(1979): 398-400; bibl.
2 cases of sudden collapse and death following instillation of PGF2alpha are analyzed, but with no explanation as to the etiology. Although some studies have shown PGF2alpha to be safer than hypertonic saline, these deaths should heighten clinicians' awareness of possible risks using the procedure.

344. Cates, Willard Jr., and Tietze, Christopher. "Standardized mortality rates associated with legal abortion: United States 1972-1975." Family Planning Perspectives 10.(1978): 109-112; bibl.
A study of the Center for Disease Control and The Alan Guttmacher Institutes' statistics for 1972-1975 affirm the authors' contention that abortions performed before the 16th week of pregnancy are safer than childbirth. This remains true when abortion-related death rates are standardized for age and race.

345. Edstrom, Karin.   "Early complications of late sequelae of induced abortion: a review of the literature." Bulletin of the World Health Organization 52.(1975): 123-139; bibl.
Author carefully reviews abortion literature in the areas of mortality and morbidity rates and techniques and complications.   Evaluation of recent literature shows wide variation in collection and presentation of research data on somatic complications of induced abortions.   There is a need for uniform definitions of complications and some uniformity in the analysis of data collected.   In addition, carefully selected control groups are needed.   Knowledge on late somatic sequelae is particularly scarce.

346. Edstrom, Karin.   "Techniques of induced abortion: their health implications and services aspects: a review of the literature." Bulletin of the World Health Organization 57.(1979): 481-497;   bibl.
Updates Edstrom's previous review (1975) of literature on abortion relating to techniques and complications.   Also evaluates literature on who should perform abortions.

347. Grimes, David A.   "Abortion facilities and the risk of death." Family Planning Perspectives 13.(Jan/Feb. l981): 30-32; bibl.
An analysis of 1974-1977 maternal deaths from abortion shows that 36 deaths were reported per 3,959,000 abortions performed, for a death-to-case rate of 0.9 deaths per l00,000 abortions.   Complications of anesthesia or analgesia were the most frequent cause of death. Deficiencies in technology, equipment, or personnel were not unique to either hospital or non-hospital facilities.

348. Hodgson, Jane E.   "Major complications of 20,248 consecutive first trimester abortions: problems of fragmented care." Advances in Planned Parenthood 9.(1975): 52-59; bibl.
The safety of outpatient first trimester abortion by suction curettage has been documented.   In this series of 20,248 procedures, the overall rate of major complications was 0.93%.   There were no maternal deaths. Complication rates can be further lowered by elimination of fragmented postabortion care.

349. Kahan, Ronald S. et al.   "The effect of legalized abortion on morbid-

ity resulting from criminal abortion."   American Journal of Obstetrics
and Gynecology 121.(January 1, 1975): 114-116;   bibl.
A surveillance system established at a large urban hospital in Atlanta,
Georgia revealed that only after 3 years of increasing numbers of legal
abortions did the number of women attempting illegal abortions
decrease.   Notes the availability of legal abortions must be sufficiently
broad to avoid the necessity for criminal abortions.

350. Lanska, M.J. et al.   "Mortality from abortion and childbirth."   JAMA
250.3 (July 15, 1983): 361-362;   bibl.
In letter, authors recommend maternal mortality figures be reported by
type of delivery (vaginal or cesarean) when compared to abortion figures,
because the maternal morality rate for cesareans is 53 times greater
than legal abortions and the statistic skews the overall figures.   In
reply, David Grimes et al state that is appropriate to use overall delivery
figures, making the mortality figure for childbirth 7 times greater than
legal abortion.

351. LeBolt, Scott A. et al.   "Mortality from abortion and childbirth: are
the populations comparable?"   Journal of the American Medical
Association 248.#2   (July 9, 1982): 188-191; bibl.
Authors calculated standardized abortion and childbirth mortality rates
betweee 1972-1978, adjusting for preexisting medical conditions.
Between 1972-1978, women were about seven times more likely to die
from childbirth than from legal abortion, with the gap increasing in more
recent years.

352. Pakter, Jean et al.   "Impact of the liberalized abortion law in New
York City on deaths associated with pregnancy: a two-year experience."
Bulletin of the New York Academy of Medicine 49.9 (September 1972):
804-818.
For the two-year period immediately following the liberalization of the
abortion law in New York City (July 1, 1970), 29 abortion-related deaths
were recorded, of which 16 followed legal abortions and 13 illegal.   For
the two-year period prior to July 1970 there were 45 abortion deaths,
all of which were in the illegal category.   The rate after legalization was
4.0 per 100,000 abortions, with the risk of fatality lowest with the
suction method (0.4 per 100,000 abortions).

353. Peterson, Herbert B. et al. "Comparative risk of death from induced abortion at less than 12 weeks' gestation performed with local versus general anesthesia." American Journal of Obstetrics and Gynecology 141.763-768;   bibl. (1981):
Using death rate statistics from the Center for Disease Control's nationwide surveillance of abortion mortality, comparisons were made among deaths resulting from various kinds of anesthesia. Adjusted death-to-case ratios reveal a higher risk of death when abortion is performed under general anesthesia than local.

354. Pike, M.C. et al. "Oral contraceptive use and early abortion as risk factors for breast cancer in young women." British Journal of Cancer 43.(1981): 72-76;   bibl.
A case-control study in Los Angeles County of 163 very young breast cancer cases (all 32 or less at diagnosis) investigated the role of oral contraceptives and abortion in relation to the disease. A first-trimester abortion before first full-term pregnancy, whether spontaneous or induced, was associated with a 2.4-fold increase in breast cancer risk.

355. Roht, Lewis H. et al. "Impact of legal abortion: redefining the maternal mortality rate." Health Services Reports 89.3 (May-June 1974): 267-273.
The maternal mortality rate has usually been measured by the ratio of deaths from all maternal causes to live births in a defined population. Researchers recommend a more accurate statistic would be all recognized conceptions, including an estimation of the gestational age at which pregnancy is concluded.

356. Sachs, Benjamin P. et al. "Reproductive mortality in the U.S." JAMA 247.20 (May 28, 1982): 2789-92;   bibl.
In a study of deaths related to reproduction (or hazards of fertility and fertility control), authors report that since 1973 all abortion-related deaths have fallen by 73%.

357. Schiffer, M.A. et al. "Mortality associated with hypertonic saline abortion." Obstetrics and Gynecology 42.(1973): 759-764; bibl.
In N.Y.C. from July 1, 1970 through June 30, 1972 there were 40,474

intraamniotic instillations of hypertonic saline for midtrimester abortion. 10 patients died. The main factors which led to deaths were complications secondary to incomplete abortion with bleeding, sepsis complications which arose from the use of other agents to shorten the instillation-abortion time and complications secondary to preexistent medical conditions.

358. Selik, Richard M. et al. "Behavioral factors contributing to abortion deaths: a new approach to mortality studies." Obstetrics and Gynecology 58.5 (November 1981): 631-635; bibl.
Mortality statistics in the U.S. from 1975-1977 were analyzed by behavioral factors (including actions by physicians, patients, communities and institutions) that increased the risk of death from abortion. The most frequent factors involved were delay in obtaining a legal abortion until 13 weeks' gestation or later, incomplete abortion, and inappropriate choice of antibiotics for septic abortion.

359. Seward, Paul N. et al. "Effect of legal abortion on the rate of septic abortion at a large county hospital." American Journal of Obstetrics and Gynecology 115.(February 1, 1973): 335-338; bibl.
The number of admissions for treatment of septic abortion in one hospital decreased from 646 to under 150 per year between 1966-1971. Legal abortion may be associated with less morbidity than illegal abortion or physicians performing the abortions may handle the initial complications.

360. Shelton, James D., and Schoenbucher, A.K. "Deaths after legally induced abortion." Public Health Reports 93.#4 (July/August 1978): 375-378; bibl.
Compares selected characteristics of Georgia residents who died after obtaining abortions in 1975. 8 of 10 deaths appeared unrelated to the abortion (accidents or other traumatic events), while 2 may possibly be related but not verified absolutely. Concludes Georgia data is consistent with national data.

361. Stewart, Gary F., and Goldstein, Phillip. "Medical and surgical complications of therapeutic abortions." Obstetrics and Gynecology

40.(October, 1972): 539-550; bibl.
Morbidity of legal abortion seems to be related to the type of procedure undertaken. Early uterine evacuation has highest morbidity in blood loss and most significant morbidity in uterine perforation. Intrauterine instillation of hypertonic saline produced morbidity from retained products of conception and from infection. Morbidity from hysterotomy or hysterectomy was associated with increased blood loss and a febrile postabortion course.

362. Stewart, Gary F., and Goldstein, Phillip. "Therapeutic abortion in California: effects on septic abortion and maternal mortality." Journal of Obstetrics and Gynecology 37.(April 1971): 510-514; bibl.
From evidence accumulated during a certain period since the implementation of the Therapeutic Abortion Act in California, both maternal mortality and incidence of septic abortions decreased significantly in the San Francisco Bay Area where a large number of therapeutic abortions was performed.

363. U.S. Department of Health, Education and Welfare. Center for Disease Control. "Comparative risks of three methods of mid-trimester abortion." Morbidity and Mortality Weekly Report 25.46 (November 26, 1976): 370-375.
Data collected from 32 institutions over a 4-year period comparing the risks of midtrimester abortion by three methods indicates that D & E was the safest, hypertonic saline the next safest, and intramniotic PGF2 the least safe.

8

Abortion Effects on Subsequent Pregnancy

364. Bracken, Michael B. "Induced abortion as a risk factor for perinatal complications: a review." Yale Journal of Biology and Medicine 51.(1978): 539-48; bibl.
Reviews literature on the influence of prior induced abortion on subsequent perinatal complications and concludes that there are some methodological difficulties in the extant literature which preclude concensus on some issues. However, the literature suggests that abortion by vacuum aspiration is not a risk factor for complications in subsequent pregnancies, while abortion by D & C may increase the risk of spontaneous abortion, low birth weight and prematurity. There is a need to examine the effect of newer abortion techniques and to clarify the impact of D & C procedures.

365. Cates, Willard Jr. "Late effects of induced abortion: hypothesis or knowledge?" Journal of Reproductive Medicine 22.(1979): 207-212; bibl.
Cautions that current data and studies do not support firm conclusions about induced abortions either causing or not causing any of the alleged long-term complications. Suggests that if late sequelae are shown to be associated with prior induced abortion, it is likely that they are related to particular abortion techniques.

366. Chung, Chin Sik et al. "Effects of Induced Abortion on Subsequent Reproductive Functions and Pregnancy Outcome: Hawaii." Papers of the East-West Population Institute. #86 (June 1983). 144 p.; bibl.
This important study details effects of induced abortion on subsequent pregnancy outcomes among women in Hawaii from 1971-1978. Clinical information was obtained from hospital records for 3,589 pairs of abor-

tion and control pregnancy groups matched on age and race of the women and on time of the event.   Comparisons revealed no differences between the abortion and nonabortion groups in overall rates of spontaneous fetal loss or in second-trimester fetal loss.   The abortion group had a slightly higher rate of fetal loss than the control group in the first trimester of pregnancy.   Although there was no significant association between induced abortion and ectopic pregnancy, use of laminaria, number of prior induced abortions or length of gestation, women with a history of postabortion infection or retained secundines had an incidence of ectopic pregnancy 5 times greater than among others in the abortion cohort. Also includes literature review and extensive statistical tables.

367. Chung, Chin Sik et al.   "Induced abortion and spontaneous fetal loss in subsequent pregnancies."   American Journal of Public Health 72.#6 (June, 1982): 548-554; bibl.
This paper is one segment of Chung's longer study ("Effects of induced abortion on subsequent reproductive functions and pregnancy outcome"). The effect of induced abortion on spontaneous pregnancy loss in subsequent pregnancies was studied through the comparison of 3,416 pairs of matched data.   Pregnancy outcome was examined in relation to abortion procedure, gestational length at the time of abortion, and number of previous abortions.   In general there was no significant association between prior induced abortion and risks of pregnancy loss.

368. Craft, Ian et al.   "Consequences of induced abortion." Lancet 1.(February 24, 1979): 437.
In a letter to the editor, authors criticize the W.H.O. Task Force Report on the Sequelae of Abortion because ot its epidemiological limitations. Suggests cervical stress at termination in the first trimester can lead to difficulties in labor.   Authors have since changed their abortion techniques.   To avoid trauma to the lower uterus and cervix, extra-amniotic prostaglandin in gel is used instead of inter-amniotic prostaglandins.

369. Daling, Janet R. et al.   "Role of induced abortion in secondary infertility."   Obstetrics and Gynecology 57.(1981): 59-61; bibl.
Medical histories of patients with secondary infertility and control cases were matched.   Women with a history of prior induced abortion did

have a slightly higher risk (1.31) of secondary infertility but the confidence interval was consistent with no association at all.   Cautions need for larger series studies.

370. Daling, Janet Roscoe.   Subsequent Pregnancy Outcome following Induced Abortion.   University of Washington: 1977.   114 p.;   bibl.
Reviews literature on the effects of induced abortion on subsequent pregnancy outcomes.   The study which follows uses sampling of over 5000 women who gave birth in Seattle,Washington from July,1972-July 1976.   Variables in the matched pair analysis included pregnancy order, marital status, socioeconomic status, prior fetal death, maternal age and religion.   In no analysis was a history of prior induced abortion significantly related to adverse pregnancy outcomes such   as low birthweight or neonatal death.   However, women with a history of induced abortion experienced higher complication rates of prolonged labor, toxemia, and   primary cesarean section.

371. Daling, Janet Roscoe, and Emanual, Irvin.   "Induced abortion and subsequent outcome of pregnancy in a series of American women."   New England Journal of Medicine 297.(December 8, 1977): 1241-1245;   bibl.
Authors studied effects of induced abortion on outcome of subsequent pregnancy in a sample of 4896 women in Seattle, Washington.   Using a matched pair analysis, they found that histories of prior induced abortions were not related to low birth weight, premature delivery, stillbirth, neonatal death, miscarriage or congenital malformations in subsequent pregnancies.

372. Harlap, Susan, and Davies, A. Michael.   "Late sequelae of induced abortion: complications and outcome of pregnancy and labor."   American Journal of   Epidemiology 102.3 (1975): 217-224;   bibl.
Measures of pregnancy outcomes were noted in a study of 11,057 West Jerusalem, Israel mothers.   The 752 mothers who reported one or more induced abortions were less likely to have a normal delivery, with increases in low birthweight, and/or minor and major fetal malformations.   There were no significant increases in stillbirth or post-neonatal death rates.

373. Hogue, Carol J. et al. "The effects of induced abortion on subsequent reproduction." Epidemiologic Reviews 4.(1982): 66-94; bibl.
A major review of over 200 reports and 150 studies. Data from the literature of the effects of induced abortion on subsequent reproduction was systematically compared and evaluated. The investigators list eight conclusions regarding the effect of prior induced abortion on subsequent reproduction, including effects on low-birth-weight, fertility, and length of gestation.

374. Hogue, Carol J. et al. "Impact of vacuum aspiration abortion on future childbearing: a review." Family Planning Perspectives 15.(1983): 119-126.
A review of studies on the impact of first-trimester induced abortion on subsequent pregnancies fails to disclose a clear pattern. Ten studies on the impact of first-trimester induced abortion by vacuum aspiration find that compared with women who carry their first pregnancy to term, women whose first pregnancy ends in induced abortion have no greater risk of low-birth-weight babies, delivering prematurely or suffering spontaneous abortions in subsequent pregnancies. No definite conclusion can be reached about the impact of multiple induced abortions.

375. Hogue, Carol J. et al. "The interactive effects of induced abortion, inter-pregnancy interval and contraceptive use on subsequent pregnancy outcome." American Journal of Epidemiology 197.(1978): 15-26; bibl.
An analysis of pregnancy records from Skopje, Yugoslavia reveals that the proportion of adverse pregnancy outcomes occurring after induced abortion does not increase for non-contraceptors. However, for the contraceptive users, proportions of adverse outcomes increased with length of pregnancy interval.

376. Hogue, Carol J. "Low birthweight subsequent to induced abortion." American Journal of Obstetrics and Gynecology 123.7 (December 1, 1975): 675-681; bibl.
Interviews were conducted with 948 Yugoslavian women whose first pregnancies were terminated by induced abortion or delivery. In a study of subsequent pregnancies, no significant differences were found between first pregnancy aborters and deliverers for subsequent conception rates, spontaneous abortions, or low birth-weight ratios.

377. Kline, Jennie et al. "Induced abortion and spontaneous abortion: no connection?" American Journal of Epidemiology 107.4 (1978): 290-8; bibl.
Reproductive histories of a consecutive series of women admitted to hospital with spontaneous abortions were compared with those of a control series of women who delivered after 28 weeks of gestation. The study showed there is no association between spontaneous abortion and prior induced abortion.

378. Levin, Ann A. et al.   "Association of induced abortion with subsequent pregnancy loss." JAMA 243.(June 27, 1980): 2495-9; bibl.
A comparison of prior pregnancy records for two groups of multigravidas demonstrated a twofold to threefold increase in the risk of first trimester spontaneous abortions for women who had had two or more prior induced abortions. No increase of pregnancy loss was detected among women with a single prior induced abortion.

379. Levin, Ann A.   "Ectopic pregnancy and prior induced abortion." American Journal of Public Health 72.(March, 1982): 253-6; bibl.
Several risk factors for ectopic pregnancy are indicated in this study. When multivariate techniques are used to control the effects of these factors simultaneously, there was no detectable increase in the risk of ectopic pregnancy for women who had had one prior induced abortion. The risk for women who had had two or more prior abortions fell from 4.0 to 2.6 and was no longer statistically significant. Under certain circumstances, a possible association exists between multiple prior induced abortions and subsequent ectopic pregnancy.

380. Linn, Shann et al. "The relationship between induced abortion and outcome of subsequent pregnancies." American Journal of Obstetrics and Gynecology 146.(1983): 136-140; bibl.
Analysis of data from 9,823 deliveries indicated that a history of one induced abortion was statistically significantly associated with first-trimester bleeding but no other untoward pregnancy events. A history of two or more induced abortions was associated with first-trimester bleeding, abnormal presentations, and premature rupture of the membranes. History of one induced abortion was not associated with the occurrence of low-birth-weight or short gestation.

381. Logrillo, Vito M. et al. "Effect of Induced Abortion on Subsequent Reproductive Function." Final report to the National Institute of Child Health and Human Development. April 18, 1980. 31 p.; bibl.
Study and control populations in New York State consisting of 20,296 women were followed up six years after live birth or abortion. Study and control groups were matched with respect to 5 variables: race, age, education, previous pregnancies and residence. Figures showed that women with previous induced abortions are more likely to abort a subsequent pregnancy than women with no history of abortion (39% vs. 12%). Authors recommend further research inconjuction with other factors such as multiple abortions, drug and alcohol use, techniques of abortion, etc.

382. Madore, Carol et al. "A study on the effects of induced abortion on subsequent pregnancy outcome." American Journal of Obstetrics and Gynecology 139.(1981): 516-521; bibl.
Records from a number of California hospitals from 1976-1978 were compared to determine the effects of previous induced abortion on subsequent pregnancy outcome. Women with a history of previous induced abortion showed a small but statistically significant increase in subsequent pregnancy failure. However, several other indicators (marital status, use of contraception, economic status and smoking) were found to be greater risk factors for an adverse outcome than a prior induced abortion.

383. Maine, Deborah. "Does abortion affect later pregnancies?" International Family Planning Perspectives 5.(1979): 22-29; bibl.
Discusses results of 7 major studies on the association of prior induced abortion with subsequent miscarriage, premature deliveries, and low-birth-weight infants. While the combined results of the studies seem to indicate that having an induced abortion may increase the risk of adverse outcome in later pregnancies, the extent of risk is not yet known.

384. Pantelakis, Stefanos N. et al. "Influence of induced and spontaneous abortion on the outcome of subsequent pregnancies." American Journal of Obstetrics and Gynecology 116.(July, l973): 799-805.
Presents results of a study of 13,242 women who were admitted for

delivery in a maternity hospital in Greece over a two-year period. Of the 8,312 women whose present pregnancy was not the first, 29% admitted one or two induced abortions. The percentage of stillbirths and premature births among the women with previous abortions was double that of the control group. Author speculates one cause for such complications might be incompetence of the internal cervical os.

385. Richardson, John A., and Dixon, G. "Effects of legal termination on subsequent pregnancy." British Medical Journal 1.(1976): 1303-4; bibl.
211 patients who had induced abortions and became pregnant again were compared with patients who were pregnant after spontaneous abortions. The overall fetal loss in the induced abortion group was 17.5% as compared with 7.5% of the spontaneous abortion group. Suggests that cervical incompetence is responsible   for the high fetal loss.

386. Roht, Lewis H., and Aoyama, Hideyasu. "Induced abortion and its sequelae: prevalence and associations with the outcome of pregnancy." International Journal of Epidemiology 2.1 (1973): 103-113; bibl.
Data obtained from the pregnancy histories of 2,476 mail survey and 614 interview survey respondents in Japan regarding the association between induced abortion and pregnancy outcome indicated that live births and pregnancies (excluding induced abortions) showed similar ratios among women who did and did not use induced abortion. Maternal age-specific analysis showed that the outcomes of pregnancies subsequent to an induced abortion were qualitatively similar to the outcomes of pregnancies in women who did not use abortion.

387. Schoenbaum, S.C. et al. "Outcome of the delivery following an induced or spontaneous abortion." American Journal of Obstetrics and Gynecology 136.(1980): 19-24; bibl.
An analysis of 5,003 singleton deliveries in 1975-76 at Boston Hospital for Women demonstrates that offspring of women with a proximate induced abortion had no higher frequency of short gestations, lower Apgar scores, or congenital malformations than those born of women with no prior loss. In contrast, offspring of secundigravidas with a proximate spontaneous abortion are a high-risk group for poor late pregnancy outcomes.

388. Slater, Paul E. et al. "The effect of method of abortion on the outcome of subsequent pregnancy." Journal of Reproductive Medicine 26.(1981): 123-138;   bibl.
A study of infants born to women following a previous induced abortion, primarily from the D & C method, showed a slight excess of low-birth-weight rate.   The data suggests that women requiring induced abortions should have them as early as possible to minimize cervical damage.

389. Trichopoulos, D. et al. "Induced abortion and secondary infertility." British Journal of Obstetrics and Gynecology 83.(1976): 645-50;   bibl.
Obstetric and gynecologic records of 83 patients with secondary infertility and 166 matched control subjects were examined to determine the role of induced abortion in the etiology of secondary infertility.   The risk of secondary infertility among women with at least one induced abortion was 3.4 times that among women without any induced or spontaneous abortions.

390. WHO Task Force on the Sequelae of Abortion.   "Gestation, birthweight, and spontaneous abortion in pregnancy after induced abortion." Lancet 1.(January   20, 1979): 142-145.
The outcome of pregnancy in 7228 women from eight European cities was studied.   In two of three city clusters there was a significantly higher risk of adverse outcome among women whose only previous pregnancy had been surgically terminated than among primigravidae or women whose only previous pregnancy had ended in live birth.   In the third city cluster in which surgical termination was nearly entirely by vacuum aspiration, induced abortion was not associated with any increased risk of adverse pregnancy outcome.

391. Wright, Charles S. et al.   "Second trimester abortion after vaginal termination of pregnancy." Lancet i.(1972): 1278-1279; bibl.
During 1971 in Queen Charlotte's Hospital in London, England, there was a tenfold increase in the number of second-trimester abortions in pregnancies which followed a vaginal termination of pregnancy, compared with all patients who delivered in the same year.   This increase suggests that temporary or permanent cervical incompetence is induced by the procedure of dilatation of the cervix during termination.

Patients who have had a vaginal termination should be judged at risk of having a second trimester abortion and should be treated for cervical incompetence.

9

Psychological Effects

392. Abernathy, Virginia. "The abortion constellation: early history and present relationships." Archives of General Psychiatry 29.(1973): 346-350; bibl.
65 married and single women who had an abortion were compared with matched controls who appeared to be effective contraceptive users. It seems that the dynamics involved in risking an unwanted pregnancy include low self-esteem, dependency, and anxiety related to unresolved incestuous overtones in the relationship with the father. Applications of these findings and theory for birth control programs requires more work.

393. Abrams, Marilyn. "Birth control use by teenagers: one and two years postabortion." Journal of Adolescent Health Care 6.3 (May 1985): 196-200.
182 postabortion adolescent respondents to a questionnaire regarding their use of birth control said that 77% of them were using an effective method of contraception. In the second year, 79% of the 106 who responded continued to use an effective contraceptive method. The opportunities for contraceptive counseling in abortion clinics may be an important factor in high postabortion birth control methods.

394. Abrams, Marilyn et al. "Post-abortion attitudes and patterns of birth control." Journal of Family Practice 9.4 (1979): 593-599; bibl.
Among 63 women questioned one year after a first trimester abortion at an outpatient clinic, over 75% had mature reasons for having chosen abortion and felt secure in their decision. They had become more responsible about contraceptive use. Over one third felt they were better able to deal with problems and had learned more about their coping capacity as a result of the abortion.

395. Adler, Nancy E.   "Abortion: a social-psychological perspective."
Journal of Social Issues 35.1 (l979): 100-119; bibl.
Evaluates abortion as a stress experience. Responses to the experience
will be a function of the nature and meaning of the pregnancy to the
woman, her defensive and coping style, and the abortion setting.
Emphasizes need to study the abortion experience as a whole rather than
in a fragmented way.

396. Adler, Nancy E.   "Emotional responses of women following
therapeutic abortion." American Journal of Orthopsychiatry 45.(1975):
446-454; bibl.
Factor analysis of post-abortion emotional responses revealed three
factors. Negative emotions split into two factors: socially and
internally-based.   Positive emotions, consitututing the third factor,
were experienced most strongly.

397. Athanasiou, R.   et al.   "Psychiatric sequelae to term birth and
induced early and late abortion: a longitudinal study." Family Planning
Perspectives 5.(1973): 227-231; bibl.
A comparative study of patients from The Johns Hopkins Hospital who
chose abortion or term birth.   The two groups were strikingly similar in
pre and post-procedure scores on self-esteem scales, emotional recovery
after hospitalization and psychosocial variables such as marital
happiness or frequency of sex. The one significant finding was a marked
improvement of effectiveness of contraception following birth or
abortion, attributed to motivation and post-pregnancy contraceptive
counseling.

398. Baluk, Ulana, and O'Neill, Patrick. "Health professionals' perceptions
of the psychological consequences of abortion." American Journal of
Community Psychology 8.1 (February 1980): 67-75; bibl.
Tests concerning depression, guilt, and state and trait anxiety were
administered to doctors, nurses and social workers, some of whom had
prior experience with abortion patients.   They were asked to complete
the tests as would a woman who had undergone an abortion the previous
day.   All three professional groups with prior experience showed extreme
depression, guilt and anxiety on the part of the patient as compared with
their own scores.   Suggests that these groups tend to think of abortion

patients as more depressed and anxious than reports of published literature indicate.

399. Beard, R.W. et al.   "King's termination study II: contraceptive practice before and after outpatient termination of pregnancy."   British Medical Journal (March 9, 1974): 418-421; bibl.
The study of a group of 360 women with first trimester pregnancies revealed that one third were ignorant about contraceptive methods.   The reliability of contraceptive methods used was found to be inversely related to neuroticism scores obtained from the Eysenck Personality Inventory.   Of 91% of the group seen three months after termination, 86% were using reliable contraceptive methods.   This satisfactory outcome is attributed to the system of counseling all women received before and after terminations.

400. Belsey, Elizabeth M. et al.   "Predictive factors in emotional response to abortion: King's termination study: IV."   Social Science & Medicine 11.2 (January 1977): 71-82; bibl.
Presents a detailed study of the emotional attitudes of a consecutive series of 300 women referred to King's College Hospital (London, England) for outpatient termination of first trimester pregnancies.   The study shows that the majority of women, regardless of whether they had any degree of distrubance before abortion, have regained their equilibrium within 3 months.   Those most likely to be disturbed had a history of instability, poor or no family ties, few friends, a poor work pattern, and failed to take contraceptive precautions.

401. Benderly, Beryl Lieff.   Thinking About Abortion.   New York: The Dial Press, l984. 204 p., bibl.
A sensitive and well-written account of the kinds of experiences a woman goes through at the time of abortion.   Chapter "Undergoing an abortion" shows in detail the various kinds of medical environments, supportive and hostile, while "The Aftermath" describes different psychological adjustments to abortion.

402. Blumberg, Bruce D. et al.   "The psychological sequelae of abortion performed for a genetic indication."   American Journal of Obstetrics and

Gynecology 122.(August 1, 1975): 799-808.
Testing and interviews were conducted with 13 families in which women had underdone abortion for a genetic defect in the fetus. The incidence of depression may be as high as 92% among the women and 82% among the men, and was greater than that usually associated with elective abortion for psychosocial indications. Most of the families would repeat their course of action and opt for abortion rather than have a defective child.

403. Bogen, Iver. "Attitudes of women who have had abortions." Journal of Sex Research 10.2 (May 1974): 97-109; bibl.
A followup study of 205 women who have had abortions indicates that women are generally not traumatized by the event. Approximately 11% of the women were sorrowful or depressed and/or had counseling or would like to have counseling. Also reports on other socioeconomic variables from questionnaire.

404. Canzano, Gail S. Unwanted Pregnancies Terminated by Induced Abortion: A Study in Unconscious Motivational Factors. Los Angeles: California School of Professional Psychology, 1984.
Study explores whether differences exist between women with planned pregnancies and women with unplanned pregnancies with respect to object loss. Results suggest a relationship between loss or separation from a significant other and ineffective contraceptive use. No differences were observed between groups with regard to borderline personality characteristics or somatic anxiety.

405. Cherazi, Shahla. "Brief communication: psychological reaction to abortion." Journal of the American Medical Women's Association 34.(July 1979): 287-288.
Notes two case studies where author worked with women on their reactions to loss as a result of abortion. States that the reaction of a woman to abortion will depend on her specific personality organization and psychopathology.

406. Cohen, Larry, and Roth, Susan. "Coping with abortion." Journal of Human Stress 10.3 (Fall 1984): 140-145.

55 patients who had undergoing a first trimester abortion were evaluated as to type of coping style.   At first testing (prior to abortion) the overall picture was of a fairly high level of anticipatory distress.   At second testing (five hours later) distress decreased markedly.   Styles of coping ranged from high approach-low avoidance to low approach-high avoidance.

407. Croghan, Leo M.   "Areas of potential psychological vulnerability in the new era of liberalized abortion."   Psychology 11.3 (August 1974): 35-44;   bibl.
Review of research of psychological sequelae of abortion notes that after the Supreme Court decision, climate will be better in which to conduct long-term studies of adverse sequelae.   Attention also needs to be paid to effects of abortion work on abortion clinic personnel.

408. Daily, Edwin F., and Nicholas, Nick.   "Use of conception control methods before pregnancies terminating in birth or a requested abortion in New York city municipal hospitals."   American Journal of Public Health 62.11 (November 1972): 1544-1545;   bibl.
A sample of patients counseled in 1971 in 14 municipal hospitals in New York showed that the younger a postpartum or abortion patient, the less likely it was that she used contraception in the past two years.   91% of those under the age of 15 and 66% of those ages 15-19 had not used contraception in the past two years.

409. David, Henry P.   "Abortion in psychological perspective."   American Journal of Orthopsychiatry 42.(1972): 61-68.
Surveys literature on psychological sequelae to induced abortion, psychological effects of denied abortion, and repeated abortion-seeking behavior, and concludes that better and more current studies need to be done before any conclusions can be reached.

410. David, Henry P. et al.   "Postpartum and postabortion psychotic reactions."   Family Planning Perspectives 13.(March/April 1982): 88-92.
Results of a study in 1975 when all women in Denmark under 50 years of age terminating an unwanted pregnancy or carrying to term were screened for admission to psychiatric hospitals within three months

after abortion or delivery. Overall findings indicate a postabortion admission rate of I2.6 admissions per I0,000 women and a postdelivery admission rate of II.9 admissions per I0,000 women.

411. Eliot, Stephen V.   The Determinants of Psychological Response to Abortion.   Yeshiva University, 1976.
Pre-abortion and post-abortion tests were given to a number of women to determine psychological response to abortion.   High psychic involvement with the fetus produced a pre-abortion stress syndrome characterized by difficulty making the decision, ambivalence, guilt and depression.   Psychic investment with the fetus was not highly predictive of post-abortion stress and depression.

412. Ewing, J. , and Rouse, B.   "Therapeutic abortion and a prior psychiatric history." American Journal of Psychiatry 130.(I973): 37-40.
A follow-up study of 126 women who received abortion on psychiatric grounds.   52 women with a history of psychiatric illness did not experience significantly more post-abortion emotional reactions than the others.   96% of the psychiatric group and 92% of the others reported that their emotional health was better or normal afterward.

413. Fingerer, Marsha E. .   "Psychological sequelae of abortion: anxiety and depression." Journal of Community Psychology 1.(April, 1973): 221-225; bibl.
Five groups of people ranging from abortion patients to postdoctoral students in psychology were given psychological tests in order to assess the degree of anxiety and depression accompanying an abortion. Analysis of the tests indicates there is no anxiety after abortion and some mild depression, possibly transient situational reaction adjustment.

414. Ford, Charles V. et al. "Abortion, is it a therapeutic procedure in psychiatry?" JAMA 218.(November 22, 1971): 1173-1178.
40 women of lower socioeconomic status who had requested abortion were studied psychiatrically and psychologically, and 30 were approved for abortion. 22 of these were seen in follow-up studies 6 months later. Statistics confirmed the clinical impression that for most women the abortion had been therapeutic.

415. Ford, Charles V. et al.   "Therapeutic abortion: who needs a psychiatrist?" <u>Obstetrics and Gynecology</u> 38.(1971): 206-213; bibl.
Clinical experience in evaluating more than 500 women for therapeutic abortion has led to the development of 10 diagnostic syndromes.   After evaluation by psychiatric social workers, patients who exhibit signs of psychosis are referred to a psychiatrist.   After abortion, counseling should be continued for patients in all diagnostic groups to help control potential problems.

416. Ford, James H.   "Mass-produced assembly-line abortion: a prime example of unethical, unscientific medicine." <u>California Medicine</u> 117.5 (1972):   80-84.
Because the incidence of psychologic sequelae associated with abortion cannot be established scientifically, elective abortion should be labeled "experimental" rather than "therapeutic."   Author thus disagrees with policies of New York State and California regarding availability of abortions, calling the process "commercialization."

417. Francke, Linda Bird. <u>The Ambivalence of Abortion</u>. New York: Random House, 1978. 261 p.
An informal account of women's experiences with abortion, stressing their psychological adjustments.   Contrasts present-day experiences with what it was like prior to legalized abortion.

418. Freeman, Ellen W.   "Influence of personality attributes on abortion experiences." <u>American Journal of Orthopsychiatry</u> 47.(July, 1977): 503-513.
Study of questionnaire of responses of women who underwent legal abortions reveals a wide range of complex emotional reactions.   Suggests that both the resolution of negative feelings post-abortion and motivation to use contraceptives are related to individual personality characteristics.

419. Friedman, Cornelia et al.   "The decision-making process and the outcome of therapeutic abortion." <u>American Journal of Psychiatry</u> 131.(December, 1974):   1332-1337.
Reviews literature on abortion and states that it and "our own clinical

experience" indicate that there is a greater likelihood of post-abortion psychiatric illness when any of the following elements are present: coercion, medical indications, concurrent severe psychiatric illness, and/or severe ambivalence.

420. Gerrard, M. "Sex guilt in abortion patients." Journal of Counseling and Clinical Psychology. 45.(1977): 708; bibl.
A measure of sex guilt was administered to women who were planning to have abortions and women who were not pregnant but sexually active. Sex guilt was found to be significantly higher for the abortion patients than for the nonpregnant group. Further research is needed to determine whether the elevated sex guilt scores are situational or represent a more generalized personality disposition.

421. Goldsmith, Alfredo et al.   "Contraception immediately post-abortion." Advances in Planned Parenthood 10.(1974): 38-44; bibl.
On the basis of published and unpublished studies of the post-abortion period, authors conclude that IUD insertion appears to be the most suitable method of contraception for women who have a low level of motivation with regard to   contraception.

422. Greenglass, Esther R.   After Abortion. Don Mills, Ontario: Longman,Canada, l976. 147 p.; bibl.
A psychological study of 188 Canadian women who received legal abortions and 83 women who did not receive abortions. One finding is that a woman's psychological adjustment after abortion cannot be understood without a full appreciation of the social context in which the abortion has taken place. Variations in adjustment due to religious and socio-economic status are also discussed.

423. Greer, H.S.   "Psychosocial consequences of therapeutic abortion: King's Termination Study III." British Journal of Psychiatry 128.(1976): 74-79; bibl.
A follow-up study of 360 women who underwent termination of first trimester pregnancies. Each patient received brief counseling before termination of the pregnancy. Questions were asked by means of a detailed, structured interview at 3 months and between 15 months and

24 months.   Outcome was assessed in terms of psychiatric symptoms, guilt feelings, adjustment in marital and other personal relationships, sexual responsiveness and work record.   Compared with ratings of psychosocial adjustment before term, significant improvement had occurred in all areas except marital adjustment where there was no change.   Adverse psychiatric and social sequelae were rare.

424. Hembree, Janice D.   Pre-Abortion Psychological Experience and its Relationship to Post-Abortion Psychological Outcome.   Gainesville, Florida: University of Florida, 1978.
Pre-abortion and post-abortion psychological variables were correlated for 54 women who obtained abortions on demand.   Difficulty in deciding to abort correlated with guilt about the abortion.   Guilt was more related to ambivalence about the abortion than a sense of moral guilt.

425. Jacques, Robert.   "Abortion and psychological trauma."   Medical Arts and Sciences 27.(1973): 52-59;   bibl.
Reviews data and current literature on psychological effects of abortion. Concludes there is minimal psychological trauma associated with therapeutic and legal abortion.   In cases where severe trauma has been encountered, it has been the result of psychological problems antecedent to the abortion.

426. Kalmar, Roberta.   Abortion: The Emotional Implications.   Dubuque, Iowa: Kendall/Hunt Pub. Co., 1977. 130 p.; bibl.
A series of concise essays on the psychological and emotional consequences of therapeutic abortion.   Also contains a series of essays on counseling for women pre and post abortion.

427. Kane, Francis J., and Lachenbruch,, P.   "Motivational factors in abortion patients."   American Journal of Psychiatry 130.3 (1973): 290-293; bibl.
99 single white women and 79 single nonpregnant women were psychologically tested.   The two groups were fairly similar as to demographic variables except for education.   The pregnant group rated themselves as more impulsive and as tending to externalize aggression. The claim of lack of information about contraception leading to

pregnancy did not prove correct.   Authors suggest that young women seeking abortion are no more neurotic as a group than nonpregnant girls their age.

428. Lask, Bryan.   "Short-term psychiatric sequelae to therapeutic termination of pregnancy."   British Journal of Psychiatry 126.(1975): 173-177.
A study of 44 patients 6 months after termination of pregnancy showed that 84% had no regrets about the termination and the psychiatric status was improved or unchanged in 89% of the cases.   Adverse outcome was usually related to the patient's environment since the operation rather than the termination itself.

429. Lawrence, William J.   "Anxiety-adjustment and other personality factors in teenage patients before and after abortion."   81st Annual Meeting of the American Psychological Association. 1973. 8: 413-414; bibl.
A comparison of anxiety scores among pregnant teenage patients (at 1st and 2nd trimester) and non-pregnant controls did not reveal significant differences.   Suggests it would have been more advisable to investigate depression rather than anxiety on the first clinic visit.   Also concludes that results are in keeping with a growing body of evidence which demonstrates that psychopathology after abortion is minimal.

430. Lazarus, Arthur.   "Psychiatric sequelae of legalized elective first trimester abortion." Journal of Psychosomatic Obstetrics and Gynecology 4.3 (Sept. 1985): 141-150; bibl.
Results of a questionnaire survey of 292 patients who underwent first trimester pregnancy terminations indicated that the predominant reaction was relief (reported by three-fourths of all patients).   Guilt and depression occurred in about 15% of patients.

431. Lebenshon, Zigmond M.   "Abortion, psychiatry and the quality of life." American Journal of Psychiatry 128.8 (February 1972): 946-951; bibl.
Reviews history of the medical profession's involvement in the abortion issue.   States that psychiatrists must address themselves to all the psychological aspects of contraception, abortion, sterilization, family

planning and population control.   Abortion should be approached "as primarily a medical   matter."

432. Lees, Robert Barry. Men and the Abortion Experience. Ann Arbor: University of Michigan, 1975.
Anxiety tests were given to 73 single men who accompanied their women partners to a Detroit abortion clinic.   Results indicated that the men were extremely anxious overall.   Anxiety was also higher for men who felt positively about their partners.   Suggests that clinics might consider counseling for male partners as a regular feature of their services.

433. Lieberman, E. James.   "The Psychological Consequences of Adolescent Pregnancy and Abortion." In Adolescent Pregnancy and Childbearing: Findings from Research. editor,   Chilman, Catherine S.(NIH Pub. No.81-2077) .   Bethesda, Md.: N.I.H., 1980. pp. 207-219.
Briefly reviews major concerns regarding psychological consequences of abortion for teenagers.   Because the chief users of legal abortion in the U.S. have been first-time pregnant, young, unmarried women, abortion service becomes a channel of contraceptive education and practice.

434. Lieh-Mak, F. et al.   "Husbands of abortion applicants: a comparison with husbands of women who complete their pregnancies."   Social Psychiatry 14.2 (April 1979): 59-64;   bibl.
Two groups of husbands of women requesting abortion and husbands of women who completed their pregnancies were compared.   The two groups differed in several respects: among them, the abortion cases were significantly older;   they had more social and economic problems;   and they tended to use unreliable contraceptive methods.

435. Maes, John L.   "The psychological antecedent and the consequences of abortion." Journal of Reproductive Medicine 8.6 (June 1972): 341-344.
Acknowledges that women who make the abortion decision have to face a difficult situation.   Stresses need for physician to treat women seeking an abortion with compassion and respect for her as a person.

436. Major, Brenda et al.   "Attributions, expectations, and coping with abortion." Journal of Personality & Social Psychology 48.3 (March, 1985): 585-599;   bibl.
A survey of 247 women undergoing first trimester abortion was completed to examine the role of three psychological factors--causal attributions, expectations for coping, and ability to find meaning. Women who engaged in more self-character blame coped significantly less well than women who engaged in less self-character blame. However, the degree to which women blamed their pregnancy on their own behavior had no impact on their coping responses. Subjects who were accompanied by partners experienced more depression following the abortion.

437. Mall, David, and Watts, Walter F., eds. Psychological Aspects of Abortion.   156 p.   Washington, D.C.: University Publications of America, 1979.
A number of essays by contributors writing from an anti-abortion point of view. Covers such topics as abortion and child abuse, pregnancy and rape, incest, and post-abortion psychoses.

438. Marder, Leon L.   "Psychiatric experience with a liberalized abortion law." American Journal of Psychiatry 126.(1970): 1230-1236.
Reviews experience with 147 patients treated under a liberalized abortion law.   Concern and proper care minimized the development of guilt, remorse and depression.   Patients generally described marked relief of symptoms and reported improvement in their relationships with others following the abortion.

439. Margolis, Alan et al.   "Contraception after abortion." Family Planning Perspectives 6.(1974): 56-60;   bibl.
303 women were interviewed after their abortion to determine contraceptive use. 93% obtained a method of contraception when the abortion was performed, and 91% were still using contraception 6 months later.   By the time of the second interview, more than one-quarter had switched from original method of contraception, the largest number being from IUD and/or pill to other (or no) method. Stresses importance of providing counseling and contraceptive choice at time of abortion.

440. Maxton-Graham, Katrina.   Pregnant by Mistake: the Stories of Seventeen Women. New York: Liveright, 1973. 435 p.
Interviews with seventeen women about their abortions (both legal and illegal) reveal a wide range of feelings and emotions.   The interviews, although edited, are fairly lengthy and are useful in providing first-hand accounts of psychological reactions to the procedures.

441. Meyerowitz, Sanford   et al.   "Induced abortion for psychiatric indications."   American Journal of Psychiatry   127.March   (1971): 1153-1160; bibl.
Women considered for induced abortion for psychiatric indications under a restrictive state law were studied over a period of seven years.   The recommendation for abortion was unrelated to a number of social variables but was associated with judged suicide risk and psychiatric diagnosis.   Most patients, both those who had abortions and those who carried the pregnancy to term were better or unchanged in overall psychosocial competence at long-range follow-up.   A small group of women who aborted were judged worse;   this group showed evidence of immediate adverse response after abortion.

442. Miller, Eva et al.   "Impact of the abortion experience on contraceptive acceptance."   Advances in Planned Parenthood 12.(1977): 15-28; bibl.
Data on sociodemographic characteristics, contraceptive methods and the abortion procedure from patients of PRETERM in Washington, D.C. were analyzed.   During the month of conception, 52% of all patients (N=5877) had not used contraception, while at follow-up 92.6% of the patients who had returned for follow-up (N=3518) were using some method of contraception.   Patients in the follow-up group generally selected a more effective contraceptive method than the one previously used.

443. Miller, Warren B.   "Psychological vulnerability to unwanted pregnancy."   Family Planning Perspectives 5.4 (Fall 1973): 199-201.
Discusses five aspects of ego psychology which may bear on the occurrence of unwanted pregnancies.   Also covers eight periods in a woman's life cycle, from puberty to menopause, in which a woman may be especially vulnerable to pregnancy, and her need for abortion services

during these times.

444.   Monsour, Karem J., and Steward, Barbara.   "Abortion and sexual behavior in college women."   American Journal of Orthopsychiatry. 43. (1973): 804-814;   bibl.
A study of 20 single women points to abortion as a procedure which brings relief from stress and resolves the crisis of unwanted pregnancy. The major effect on their sexual attitudes and behavior was to increase their own sense of future caution and acceptance of responsibility for their own behavior.

445. Moseley, D.T. et al.   "Psychological factors that predict reactions to abortion."   Journal of Clinical Psychology 37. (April, 1981): 276-279; bibl. Investigation of demographic and psychological factors in 62 women who had first trimester abortions.   Indicates that the most important determinant of the woman's psychological adjustment to abortion is the perceived amount of support from the woman's significant others. Suggests new psychological research needs to be made in view of the Supreme Court decision of l973.

446. Niswander, Kenneth   et al.   "Psychological reaction to therapeutic abortion,II: objective response."   American Journal of Obstetrics and Gynecology 114. September,1972 (1972): 29-33.
The Minnesota Multiphasic Inventory test was administered to 65 abortion patients and 20 maternity patients.   Postoperatively, the abortion patients were less "normal" in over-all adjustment, anxiety depression and impulsivity.   The abortion group showed an improvement in psychological state 6 months after abortion except in impulsivity. [Niswander's earlier study, "Psychological reaction to therapeutic abortion: I subjective patient response"(Obstetrics and gynecology 29:702-706, l967), explores personal reactions from patients and elicits comments. Few women in the group regretted having the abortion.   Minor doubts were fairly common but nearly always accompanied by the expressed belief that the decision to abort had been a good one.   It is useful to compare   Niswander's 1967 study with the 1972 one].

447. Oppel, Warren et al.   "Contraceptive antecedents to early and late

therapeutic abortions." American Journal of Public Health 62.6 (June, 1972): 824-827.
Authors studied contraceptive antecedents for a group of 100 early abortion patients and 100 late abortion patients. The early abortion group had a higher proportion of women who used contraception prior to pregnancy. The two groups did not differ in regard to contraceptive knowledge nor in regard to sexual experience. Concludes that less effort should be spent on contraceptive educational programs per se but more counseling needs to be done to help these women overcome their past inhibitions about the use of contraceptives. In addition, follow-up studies should be done on repeat pregnancy and on subsequent social relationships as well as on the medical sequelae of abortion.

448. Ory, Howard W. et al. Making Choices: Evaluating the Health Risks and Benefits of Birth Control Methods. New York: The Alan Guttmacher Institute, 1983. 72 p; bibl.
Using clear charts, statistically outlines various methods of contraception and their relative risks. Also delineates accessibility of types of contraception, including abortion. Section"misperceptions and open questions" provides factual information on common questions about contraceptive methods.

449. Osofsky, Joy D. , and Osofsky, Howard J. "Psychological reaction of patients to legalized abortion." American Journal of Orthopsychiatry 42.1 (1972): 48-60.
Reviews literature from diverse sources in the U.S. and abroad and concludes that abortion is accompanied by few objective psychological sequelae. Present study shows that relief and happiness have been the dominant moods post-abortion. Recommends that more objective studies be done in order to offer additional and better preventative and therapeutic services.

450. Pare, C.M.B. , and Raven, H. . "Psychiatric sequelae to therapeutic abortion." Lancet i.7648 (1970): 635-637.
321 patients in St. Bartholomew's Hospital in London were referred for follow-up after consideration of termination of pregnancy. Termination of pregnancy caused little disturbance provided the patient wanted the abortion; continuation of pregnancy on occasion led to serious

psychiatric disability, and a third of the mothers who kept their babies showed evidence of resenting them.

451. Pasnau, Robert O.   "Psychiatric complications of therapeutic abortion." Obstetrics and Gynecology 40.(1972): 252-256.
Reviews literature regarding the psychiatric complications of induced abortion. Notes that myths of serious emotional sequelae were exploded by the reevaluation of the older reports and undertaking of new studies. Most normal women were found to react to abortions with mild feelings of depression without serious after-effects.

452. Payne, E.D.   et al.   "Outcome following therapeutic abortion." Archives of General Psychiatry 33. (June, 1976): 725-733.
Psychological outcome of abortion was studied in 102 patients.   Five measured effects--anxiety, depression, guilt, anger, and shame--were significantly lower six months after the preabortion period.   Data suggests that women most vulnerable to conflict are those who are single and nulliparous or who have emotional problems and/or conflicts with lovers or mother.

453. Perez-Reyes, M.   et al.   "Follow-up after therapeutic abortion in early adolescence." Archives of General Psychiatry 28.(1973): 120-126; bibl.
Distinguishes among 3 types of adolescent pregnant girls: 1) very young, inexperienced, passive; 2) somewhat older, more experienced, sexually experimentive;   3) has a history of emotional problems.   Suggests different kind of psychiatric follow-up is needed for each type of girl.

454. Potter, Robert G.   "Additional births averted when abortion is added to contraception." Studies in Family Planning 3.(April 1972): 54-59; bibl.
A study of two cohorts in Taiwan revealed than when repeated abortion is added to contraception, the additional births averted per abortion depend primarily on the frequency and caliber of accompanying contraception.   The age of the women at the time of abortion and its timing within pregnancy tend to be secondary factors.

455. Resnik, H.L.P., and Wittlin, Byron J. "Abortion and suicidal behaviors: observations on the concept of endangering the mental health of the mother." Mental Hygiene 55.(January 1970): 10-20; bibl.
General mental health guidelines are suggested for assisting the non-psychiatric physician in arriving at his/her decision regarding abortion for the patient. In the absence of a legal action (1970), such guidelines are all based upon the concept of "endangering the mental health of the mother."

456. Rifkin, John Robert. Relationships and Abortion.   Boulder: University of Colorado, 1983.   171 p.
Tests administered to couples in which the woman was undergoing a first trimester abortion found that couples in relationships with higher levels of commitment at time of abortion were likely to be more satisfied at the three-month follow-up. Slightly less than half of the females had support from their friends, while only 27% of the men had this same kind of support, which underscores the need for counseling of both partners.

457. Robbins, J.H. "Objective vs. subjective responses to abortion." Journal of Consulting and Clinical Psychology 47.(1979): 994-995.
Two tests, one objective and one subjective ("Do you ever regret having an abortion?") were given to 41 unmarried women who had abortions. Analysis of convariance indicated no relation between the objective and subjective indicators.

458. Robbins, James M. "Out of-wedlock abortion and delivery: the importance of the male partner." Social Problems 31.3 (February 1984): 334-350; bibl.
Research on the relationships of single women who had abortions reveal the following: 1) women with partners who are more economically secure are likely to abort the first pregnancy; 2)women are less likely to be in love with partners than delivering women; 3)relationships are no more likely to end than the relationships of delivering women; 4)relationships that are stronger after abortion seem to be associated with greater feelings of regret. Concludes importance of male partner as an influence on a woman's reaction to abortion is not as strong as has been assumed in previous literature.

459. Robbins, James M., and DeLamater, John D. "Support from significant others and loneliness following induced abortion." Social Psychiatry 20.2 (1985): 92-99.
A sampling of women who received abortions in 1973-1974 at a University Medical Center was studied to investigate the relationship between support and loneliness following abortion. One quarter of the women sampled reported feeling lonely at least half of the time one week after the experience. The male partner had a much greater effect as protection against feelings of loneliness than parents or other friends and relatives.

460. Rothstein, Arden A. "Adolescent males, fatherhood, and abortion." Journal of Youth and Adolescence 7.2 (June 1978): 203-214; bibl.
Adolescent (N=35) and adult males (N=25) who accompanied their partners to an abortion clinic were questioned regarding their sense of fatherliness. A comparison of the two groups showed that adolescents may experience issues universal to the development of fatherhood but with the variant of a concern over autonomous action.

461. Schilling, Lee H. "Postcoital contraception: awareness of the existence of postcoital contraception among students who have had a therapeutic abortion." Journal of American College Health 32.6 (June 1984): 244-246; bibl.
In a survey of women attending a women's health clinic (N= 437), of the 41% having a therapeutic abortion, 84.9% of those were not aware of PCC (postcoital contraception). Ignorance of the procedure appears to be the main reason for its underutilization.

462. Selstad, Georgiana M. et al. "Predicting contraceptive use in postabortion patients." American Journal of Public Health 65.7 (1975): 708-13; bibl.
83 post-abortion patients were studied for methods of contraception usage. The kind of person most likely to be a successful contraceptor following her abortion is a person who approves of premarital sexual activity and contraception and whose girl friends and sexual partners approve of premarital sexual activity. Authors state that any therapeutic abortion service that does not offer extensive family planning counseling services at the time of abortion is negligent.

463. Senay, Edward C.   "Therapeutic abortion: clinical aspects."   <u>Archives of General Psychiatry</u> 23. (November 1970): 408-415.
Discusses the psychiatrist's role in the abortion process.   Admits difficulty of attempting to distinguish between patients who have personal needs for wanting an abortion and those who are acting upon the wishes of others.   Maintains that in the absence of a "rational legal system" the psychiatrist is bound ethically to help patients who seek abortions.

464. Shalaby, Lynn M.   <u>How Women Feel about Abortion: Psychological, Attitudinal and Physical Effects of Legal Abortion</u>. Iowa City, Iowa: University of Iowa, 1975. 171 p.; bibl.
127 women at an abortion clinic and 106 women at a hospital clinic answered questionnaires regarding their abortion experiences.   A second follow-up questionnaire was sent to 54 of the abortion clinic group. Findings included: 1) abortion is a painful physical procedure for many women; 2) being accompanied to the procedure by a supportive person is seen as very important;   3) in general women experience abortion positively.

465. Shostak, Arthur B., and McLouth, Gary.   <u>Men and Abortion: Losses, Lessons and Love</u>. New York: Praeger, 1984. 350 p.; bibl.
A valuable, lengthy compendium of information about the subject of men's reactions to their partners' abortions.   Authors used responses from 1,000 questionnaires given to men accompanying women undergoing abortions at clinics. Profiles of individual men provide first-hand accounts of their experiences.   Chapters cover before the abortion, clinic day, repeaters, and abortion aftermath and counseling.   Appendices and charts contain useful statistical data.

466. Shusterman, Lisa R.   "Predicting the psychological consequences of abortion." <u>Social Science and Medicine</u> 13A.6 (1979): 683-689; bibl.
Pre-abortion interviews were given to 345 women and 289 follow-up interviews.   Almost 75% of the women were employed or attending school.   Many of the women belonged to conservative or fundamentalist religions.   Two major types of women were found-- young, single, primagravidae and older, multiparous women.   Few women suffered negative psychological after-effects.

467. Smith, Elizabeth M.   "A follow-up study of women who request abortion."   American Journal of Orthopsychiatry 43.(July, 1973): 574-585; bibl.
A study of 80 women who obtained abortions.   The women were interviewed prior to the abortion and one to two years later. 78% did not experience psychological reactions and 90% denied psychological changes at the time of follow-up.   Author states there is need for further systematic studies of abortion and methods for predicting at-risk women for post-abortion reactions.

468. Smith, Mark Randall.   How Men who Accompany Women to an Abortion Service Perceive the Impact of Abortion upon Their Relationship and Themselves. Iowa City: University of Iowa, 1979. 249 p.; bibl.
100 men who accompanied women to an abortion clinic were interviewed about their experiences with abortion.   The importance of the abortion to the lives of these men was found to be equal to that reported by women. The number of men and women experiencing difficulty with the decision to terminate was equivalent. These findings support the concept of abortion as being a product of a relationship process and therefore should not be treated as a "woman' problem."

469. Speckhard, Annie Catherine.   The Psycho-Social Aspects of Stress Following Abortion. Minneapolis, Minn.: University of Minnesota, 1985. 217 p.
In-depth interviews with 30 women having high stress abortion experiences reveal predominant emotional and behavioral reactions. Type of abortion is related to stress symptoms, with saline procedure having the highest degree of immediate stress.   Family relations and social systems were important factors in how the woman defined the abortion and her reactions to it.

470. Theobald, Ellen M.   A Post-Abortion Study and Attitude Comparison of Women who had and not Given Birth to Living Children. International University, 1985. 283 p.
Results from a study of abortion patients (women who had given birth and women who had not given birth) indicated that the two groups do not differ significantly in post-abortion attitudes towards abortion and abortion-related concepts.   The two groups did show differences in

demographics and life and abortion-related experiences.

471. Tietze, Christopher et al. Birth Control and Abortion. New York: MSS Information Corporation, 1972. 289 p.
Section "Psychiatric aspects of abortion" contains three articles on abortion and the psychiatrist, social, psychiatric and psychoanalytic perspectives and psychodynamic effects of abortion.

472. Todd,N.A.   "Follow-up of patients recommended for therapeutic abortion." British Journal of Psychiatry 120.(1972): 645-649.
63 of 69 patients (or 91.3%) who had received abortions reported no adverse sequelae to the procedure. The remaining patients reported reactions ranging from depression to hypochondria.

473. Wallerstein, Judith S. et al. "Psychosocial sequelae of therapeutic abortion in young unmarried women." Archives of General Psychiatry 27.(1972): 828-832; bibl.
Post-abortion studies were completed of 19 unmarried women in middle and late adolescence.   At interviews conducted at 5-7 months postabortion, the women revealed a wide range of reactions. Half were doing well without real psychic disruption, while the other half exhibited signs of poor adjustment.

474. Walter, George S.   "Psychologic and emotional consequences of elective abortion." Obstetrics and Gynecology 36.(1970): 483-487.
Reviews literature on psychiatric sequelae of induced abortion and concludes that legal abortion can be performed without fear of severe psychic harm to the woman. According to the literature, psychological consequences may fall into one of these categories: l) guilt 2) disturbance of relationship with opposite sex 3) harmful effects upon others in the family unit. Since these consequences could also come as a result of pregnancy without abortion, author concludes there is a pressing need for baseline studies on the prevelance of psychologic disabilities resulting from other outcomes of pregnancy.

475. West, N.D. "Psychological impact of abortion." AORN Journal

17.(March 1973):132-138;   bibl.
Notes need for controlled studies on the psychological impact of abortion which cover individuals in both urban and rural areas and which also cover long-term follow-up evaluations.   In addition, studies should determine the impact of abortion on people other than the pregnant woman, including the man involved,   physicians, and the abortion clinic staff.

476. Westoff, Charles F. et al.   "Abortions preventable by contraceptive practice." Family Planning Perspectives 13.5 (September/October 1981): 218-23;   bibl.
A study of abortion patients in Illinois clinics (N=4,133) showed that more than one half the sample used no method of contraception at the time of pregnancy.   An estimated 70% of abortions could be averted if all women at risk were to use the pill or the IUD.   However, because there are large numbers of women for whom use of these methods is contraindicated, the development of new, safer effective contraceptive methods and better education seems to be the way to reduce the number of abortions.

477. Whittington, H.   "Evaluation of therapeutic abortion as an element of preventative psychiatry." American Journal of Psychiatry 126.9 (1970): 1224-1229;   bibl.
Reports of psychiatric literature show that women who had undergone therapeutic abortions were content and mentally healthy afterwards. Lack of studies predicting which women might become mentally ill if denied abortion means that the 1970 practice of the "abortion committee decision" should be changed to decision-making process between a woman and her physician.   Author argues for change in "legislative therapeutic abortion procedures."

478. Williams, Jean Morton, and Hindell, Keith.   Abortion and Contraception: A Study of Patients' Attitudes.   Broadsheet #536 March 1972 . London: P.E.P., 1972.   62 p.
A study of 50 women in England explores the abortion decision, attitudes to the abortion, sexual behavior and contraceptive usage.   Concludes there is a need for a more comprehensive survey of abortion patients using a large, representative sample as well as follow-up studies.

10

Psychosocial Aspects

479. Andres, David et al. "Selected psychosocial characteristics of males: their relationship to contraceptive use and abortion." Personality and Social Psychology Bulletin 9.3 (September 1983): 387-396; bibl.
111 men were compared on personality characteristics and attitudes towards contraception and their partners. Men in the survey had partners who were either receiving a first trimester abortion or contraception. Men in the aborter group had more conservative views towards sex and contraceptive practices and relatively low rates of coitus. It is likely that men who have a low rate of coitus will be less able to predict and prepare adequately for sexual intercourse.

480. Bauman, Karl E. et al. "Legal abortions and trends in age-specific marriage rates." American Journal of Public Health 67.(1977): 52-53; bibl.
Correlations among various data measures suggest there may be a causal relationship between legal abortions and age-specific marriage rates. Cautions need for further study on hypothesis that some marriages are being delayed by legal abortions.

481. Bauman, Karl E. et al. "The relationship between legal abortion and marriage." Social Biology 22.(Summer 1975): 117-124; bibl.
Analyzes the relationship between legal abortion and trends in the crude marriage rate among states in the U.S. Data suggests there is an association between legal abortion and changes among crude marriage rates for the states with the highest abortion-birth ratios. If there is a causal relationship, statistically it takes 9-10 legal abortions for the unmarried to delay a marriage one year.

482. Cates, Willard Jr.   "Adolescent abortions in the United States."
Journal of Adolescent Health Care 1.(September, 1980): 18-25; bibl.
Teenagers account for about 17% of the population of childbearing women
but about 33% of all abortions.   The most important variable affecting
teenagers is that the procedures are performed significantly later in
pregnancy.   After adjusting for this factor, teenagers have lower
morbidity and mortality rates than do older women.   The availability of
legal abortion has been associated with increased use of contraceptives
by teenagers.

483. David, Henry P. et al. Abortion in Psychosocial Perspective: Trends
in Transnational Research. New York: Springer Publishing Company, 1978.
334 p.; bibl.
Studies abortion from a psychosocial perspective, considering research
experience gained in selected countries of Africa, Asia, Europe and North
and South America.

484. David, Henry P.   "Abortion: public health concerns and needed
psychosocial research."   American Journal of Public Health 61.(March
1971): 510-516; bibl.
Current (1971) high mortality and morbidity statistics for illegal
abortions   create   overburdened   hospital   bed   utilization   and
disproportionately high share of medical cost budgeting.   Improved
outpatient techniques and the possible use of prostaglandins offer
promise for future.   Needed psychosocial research includes studies of
effective contraceptive practice and repeated abortion-seeking behavior.

485. Deutsch, Marjorie B.   Personality Factors, Self-Concept, and Family
Variables Related to First Time and Repeat Abortion- Seeking Behavior in
Adolescent Women.   Washington, D.C.: American University, 1982.   124 p.
Results of a study of 96 white, middle or upper-middle class adolescents
provide a profile of the adolescent most at risk to become a multiple
abortee.   Among other personality/family dynamics correlating with
repeat abortions were: parents' marital conflict; peripheral father;
psychological instability and low self-concept.

486. Falk, Ruth et al. "Personality factors related to black teenage

pregnancy and abortion." <u>Psychology of Women Quarterly</u> 5.5, suppl. (1981): 737-746;   bibl.
The California Psychological Inventory (CPI) was administered to black adolescents who applied for therapeutic abortions (N=48), 55 who planned to have their babies(Terms) and 67 who were not pregnant.   Of the three groups, the Terms scored lowest in sociability and had the most difficulty thinking for themselves and are least accepting of themselves.   Data suggests Term women feel some void and are attempting to fill it up by having a child.   The abortion women do not have these psychological needs.   Results do not support the hope of researchers that the women deciding to have their babies would be the most mature and psychologically prepared for the role of mother.

487. Handy, Jocelyn A.   "Psychological and social aspects of induced abortion." <u>British Journal of Clinical Psychology</u> 21.1 (February 1982): 29-41;   bibl.
Author reviews literature concerning psychosocial aspects of induced abortion.   Covers the social and legal context, characteristics of women seeking abortion,contraceptive use, pre-abortion counseling, effect of method of abortion on psychological consequences and results of refused abortion.

488. Hendricks, Leo E.   "Unmarried black adolescent fathers' attitudes toward abortion, contraception, and sexuality: a preliminary report." <u>Journal of Adolescent Health Care</u> 2.3 (March 1982): 199-203.
In a limited survey of black adolescent fathers, a majority of the number indicated that, if they were responsible for the pregnancy, they would not want the girl to have an abortion.   Employed young fathers who completed 12 or more years of school were most likely to be opposed to abortion.

489. Henshaw, Stanley K. et al.   "A portrait of American women who obtain abortions." <u>Family Planning Perspectives</u> 17.2 (March/April 1985): 90-96;   bibl.
In 1981 most abortions were obtained by young women, unmarried women and white women and were performed in the first eight weeks following the last menstrual period.   The percentage of abortions that are repeat procedures has increased, representing more than one-third of all

abortions.

490. Horobin, Gordon, ed. Experience with Abortion: A Case Study of
North-East Scotland. New York: Cambridge University Press, 1973. 379
p.; bibl.
A thorough case-study of a relatively homogeneous and static population
in North-East Scotland. Study involves a variety of disciplines including
obstetrics, gynecology, psychiatry and sociology. Covers circumstances
surrounding an unwanted pregnancy, the reasons for a decision to seek an
abortion, factors which influence the abortion decision and psychological
and physical characteristics before and after the decision.

491. Illsley, Raymond, and Hall, Marion H. "Psychosocial aspects of
abortion: a review of issues and needed research." Bulletin of the World
Health Organization 53.(1976): 83-106; bibl.
A detailed review of the literature on the psychosocial aspects of
abortion shows that individual publications must be interpreted in
relation to the cultural constraints in a particular society at a particular
time. In addition, interpretations of the effects of an abortion will be
made with attention to status and availability of abortion alternatives.
Authors recommend descriptive research on populations of women in
different cultures be made and compared.

492. Kay, Clifford R., and Frank, Peter I. "Characteristics of women
recruited to a long-term study of the sequelae of induced abortion."
Journal of the Royal College of General Practitioners 31.(August 1981):
473-477; bibl.
This large-scale study of abortion cases (N=6,349) and controls
(N=8,132) showed that there was an excess of cases under 16 years and
over 35 years of age. In the control group, there was an excess of
married women and a significantly higher percentage of women whose
education had been completed under the age of 17. Other factors were
also examined, such as previous pregnancies, previous medical history,
and cigarette consumption.

493. "Legal abortion reduces out-of-wedlock births." Family Planning
Perspectives 7.1 (January/February 1975): 11-12.

Analyzes two studies which indicate that legal abortion has made a significant contribution to the reduction of illegitimate fertility in states where abortion is legal and readily available.   Data indicates that well over one half of all   legal abortions in the U.S. in 1971 were replacements for illegal abortions.

494. McCormick, E. Patricia.   Attitudes Towards Abortion. Lexington, Mass.: Lexington Books, 1975.   158 p.
A lengthy, detailed study of 200 women who had undergone abortion. Focus is on attitudes toward abortion and not the abortion behavior of the population studied.   Explores questions related to contraceptive use, religion, number of siblings, social class, marital status, parity and future child desired.

495. McCormick, E. Patricia et al.   "Psychosocial aspects of fertility regulation." In Handbook of Sexology., eds. Money, John, and Musaph, Herman. New York: Elsevier North-Holland, Inc., 1977.   pp. 621-653; bibl. Divides psychosocial aspects of contraception into three by fertility career stages: adolescence, young adult, and the later years.   Suggests priority for social science research is the couple and that populations for study be defined on the biopsychological dimension of fertility career stages.

496. Olson, Lucy.   "Social and psychological correlates of pregnancy resolution among adolescent women: a review." American Journal of Orthopsychiatry   50.3 (July 1980): 432-445; bibl.
Comprehensively reviews literature on pregnancy resolution among adolescent women and suggests that adolescent women do not constitute a "special population" with distinctive psychosocial features.   However, there are significant variables, among them: 1) white women obtain abortions at about nine times the rate of black women 2) women who seek abortions appear to have higher educational and occupational aspirations than do their term counterparts.

497. Shelton, James D.   "Very young adolescent women in Georgia: Has abortion or contraception lowered their fertility?" American Journal of Public Health 67.(1977): 616-620; bibl.

Increased access to induced abortion following the 1973 Supreme Court decision appears to be responsible for the decline in birth rate in Georgia for women under 14, rather than efforts to provide contraception for this age group.

498. Shusterman, Lisa R.   "The psychosocial factors of the abortion experience: a critical review." Psychology of Women Quarterly 1.1 (Fall 1976): 79-106.
Reviews the quality of research on the psychosocial factors of abortion. Evaluates statistical studies on women receiving therapeutic abortions as generally unreliable, while statistics on women receiving legal abortions are highly reliable.   The literature on the psychological effects of abortion is quite contradictory;   many conclude that there are mild or no consequences and some conclude that the consequences vary with the other factors.

499. Sklar, June, and Berkov, Beth.   "Abortion, illegitimacy and the American birth rate." Science 185.(September 13, 1974): 909-915;   bibl.
Using statistics for legal abortions and illegitimate births, authors estimated that if legalized abortion had not been available in 1971 (in certain states), an additional 39,000 illegitimate babies and 28,000 legitimate babies would have been born in the U.S.   In addition to preventing the illegitimate births, the legalization of abortion appears to have reduced the incidence of pregnancy-related marriages.

500. Zimmerman, Mary K. Passage through Abortion: the Personal and Social Reality of Women's Experiences. Praeger Special Studies in U.S. Economic, Social, and Political Issues.   New York: Praeger Publisher, 1977. 222 p.; bibl.
After reviewing previous social and psychological studies of abortion, author explains methodology.   Her studied community of 165,000 (here called Midville) is conservative and relatively prosperous.   Zimmerman interviewed 40 women who had sought abortions, and their in-depth responses are reported.   Author stresses the importance of viewing the abortion experience as a pattern of inter-related events rather than a static experience.   In addition, she notes the significance of exploring the abortion as an action which has taken place within a dynamic social structure involving relationships with partner, family, and friends.

Author Index

Abbott, Mildred I., 67
Abernathy, Virginia, 392
Abrams, Marilyn, 393-94
Addelson, Frances, 297
Adler, Nancy E., 395-96
Allen, Doris, 69-70
Allgeier, A.R., 134
American College of Obstetricians
  and Gynecologists, 71
American Public Health
  Association, 72
Amy, J.J., 1
Anderson, G.G., 220
Andolsek, L., 279
Andres, David, 479
Andrikopoulos, Bonnie, 30
Anwyl, J.H., 298
Aoyama, Hideyasu, 386
Arnstein, Helene S., 2
Asher, John D., 299
Ashton, J.R., 135-36
Athanasiou, R., 397
Atienza, Milagros F., 221

Ballard, Charles A., 239
Baluk, Ulana, 398

Barr, Maxwell M., 222
Barr, Samuel J., 137
Bauer, Herbert, 300
Bauman, Karl E., 480-1
Beard, R.W., 399
Becker, Marshall H., 104-6
Belsey, Elizabeth M., 400
Bendel, Richard P., 223
Benderly, Beryl L., 401
Benditt, John, 194
Berger, G.S., 195, 224-25
Bergstrom, Sune, 234
Beric, B., 226
Berkov, Beth, 499
Bernstein, Norman R., 301
Bluett, Desmond G., 196
Bluford, Robert Jr., 3
Blumberg, Bruce D., 402
Blumenfield, Michael, 138
Bogen, Iver, 403
Bolognese, Roland J., 4
Bongaarts, John, 227
Borell, U., 226
Boston Women's Health Book
  Collective, 5
Bourne, Judith P., 73
Bozorgi, Nader, 74

Bracken, Michael B., 6,
    139-43, 185, 302, 364
Branch, Benjamin N., 75
Brashear, Diane B., 303
Braude, Marjorie, 7
Brenner, William E., 197,
    229-30
Brewer, Colin, 144-45
Buckle, A.E.R., 231
Buckles, Nancy B., 304
Burkman, Ronald T., 232
Burnell, George M., 305
Burnett, L.S., 198-99
Burr, Winthrop A., 146
Butler, J. Douglas, 8
Bygdeman, M., 233-34

Cadesky, K.I., 235
Callahan, Daniel, 9
Canzano, Gail S., 404
Carmen, Arlene, 306
Cates, Willard Jr., 10-11,
    76, 236-37, 252, 282,
    336-44, 365, 482
Caudle, Jan, 81
Char, Walter F., 77, 103
Chaudry, Susan L., 200
Cherazi, Shahla, 405
Chez, Ronald A., 238
Chilman, Catherine S., 12
Chung, Chin Sik, 366-67
CIBA Foundation Symposium, 13
Cohen, Larry, 406
Columbia University School of
    Social Work, 307
Copeland, Pamela, 319
Corlett, Robert C., 239
Cornelio, David A., 147
Corrigan, Billie, 91
Corsaro, Maria, 14

Corson, Stephen L., 201
Cotroneo, Margaret, 308
Crabtree, Pamela Hinckley, 148
Craft, Ian, 368
Croghan, Leo M., 407
Culliton, Barbara J., 15

Daily, Edwin F., 408
Daling, Janet Roscoe, 369-71
Danon, Ardis H., 78
Dauber, Bonnie, 309
David, Henry P.,
    409-10, 469-70, 483-84
Davies, A. Michael, 372
Davis, Geoffrey, 241
DeLamater, John D., 459
Denes, Magda, 16
Denney, Myron K., 17
Deutsch, Marjorie B., 485
Diagram Group, 202
Diamond, Milton, 149
Dixon, G., 385
Dornblaser, Carole, 18
Dunlop, Joyce L., 310
Dunn, Patricia, 18

Ebon, Martin, 19
Edelman, D.A., 230, 243
Edstrom, Karin, 345-46
Eisen, Marvin, 150
Eliot, Stephen V., 411
Elms, Alan C., 171
Emanual, Irvin, 371
Erlien, Marla, 20
Ewing, J., 412

Fairchild, Ellen, 79
Falk, Ruth, 486

Federation of Feminist Women's
  Health Centers, 204
Felton, Gerald, 80
Fielding, W.L., 151
Filshie, G.M., 261
Fingerer, Marsha E., 413
Finks, Arnold A., 244
Fischer, Edward H., 81
Fleming, Alice, 205
Ford, Charles V., 414-15
Ford, James H., 416
Fortney, Judith A., 245
Francke, Linda Bird, 417
Francome, Colin, 21
Frank, Peter I., 492
Freeman, Ellen W., 153-54, 418
Freiman, S.M., 130
Friedlander, Myrna L., 155
Friedman, Cornelia, 419

Gardner, Joy, 22
Gardner, R.F.R., 23
Gedan, Sharon, 311
Gerrard, M., 420
Gibb, Gerald D., 156-57, 312
Gill, Robin, 313
Gilligan, Carol, 158
Golditch, Ira M., 246
Goldmann, Alice, 82
Goldsmith, Alfredo, 421
Goldsmith, Sadja, 83, 208, 247
Goldstein, Michael S., 84
Goldstein, Phillip, 84, 361-62
Gordon, Robert H., 314
Granger, Bruce, 180
Greenglass, Esther R., 422
Greenhalf, J.O., 248
Greer, H.S., 423
Grimes, David A., 249-52, 338,
  347

Grimm, James W., 89
Group for the Advancement of
  Psychiatry, 159
Gutknecht, G.D., 253, 287
Guttmacher, Alan F., 24

Hafez, E.S.E., 25
Hale, Ralph W., 254
Hall, Marion H., 491
Hall, Robert E., 26, 85
Handy, Jocelyn A., 487
Hare, M.J., 315
Harlap, Susan, 372
Harper, Mary, 86
Hart, Thomas M., 87
Hausknecht, Richard U., 88
Hembree, Janice D., 424
Hendershot, Gerry E., 89
Hendin, David, 27
Hendricks, Leo E., 488
Henshaw, Stanley K., 28, 489
Hern, Warren M., 29-30,
  90-91, 206, 255
Heywood, Jane, 315
Hilgers, Thomas W., 31
Hindell, Keith, 478
Hinman, Alan R., 289
Hodari, A.A., 256
Hodgson, Jane E., 32, 257-58,
  348
Hogue, Carol J., 373-76
Holtrop, Hugh R., 259
Horobin, Gordon, 490
Horvitz, Diana F., 62
Howe, Barbara, 160

Ide, Arthur F., 33
Illsley, Raymond, 491
Imber, Jonathan B., 92

Institute of Medicine of the
  National Academy of Sciences,
  34
Irani, Katy R., 260

Jacobssen, L.B., 161
Jacques, Robert, 425
Jekel, James F., 162
Joffe, Carole, 316
Johnstone, F.D., 163
Jordaan, Harold V., 343
Joseph, Carol, 164
Joy, Stephany S., 317

Kahan, Ronald S., 349
Kahn-Edrington, Marla, 318
Kalmar, Roberta, 426
Kaltreider, Nancy B., 165-66
Kane, Francis J., 94, 427
Karim, S.M.M., 261
Karman, Harvey, 95, 262, 284
Kasl, Stanislav V., 142
Kay, Clifford R., 492
Keirse, Marc J.N.C., 263
Keith, Louis, 96
Keith, Louis G., 36
Keller, Christa, 319
Kennedy, Florence, 54
Kerenyi, Thomas D., 167, 264
Kessel, Elton, 265
Kessler, Kenneth, 97
King, Theodore M., 207
Kleinman, Ronald L., 37
Kline, Jennie, 377
Korzeniowsky, Carole, 14
Krasner, Barbara R., 308
Kreutner, A. Karen, 267
Kummer, Jerome M., 320

Lachenbruch, P., 427
Landy, Uta, 18
Lane Committee, 38
Lanska, M.J., 350
Lask, Bryan, 428
Lauersen, Niels H., 266
Laufe, Leonard E., 267
Lawrence, William J., 429
Lazarus, Arthur, 430
Leach, Judith, 168
Lebenshon, Zigmond M., 431
LeBolt, Scott A., 351
Lees, Robert Barry, 432
Legge, Jerome S., 39
Levin, Ann A., 378-79
Lewis, Stella C., 268
Lewit, Sarah, 40, 216, 269-70
Lieberman, E. James, 433
Lieh-Mak, F., 434
Lincoln, Elizabeth, 169
Linn, Shann, 380
Lodl, Karen M., 321
Logrillo, Vito M., 381
LoSciuto, Leonard A., 98
Loung, K.C., 271
Lubman, Alison J., 322
Luker, Kristin, 170
Luscutoff, Sidney A., 171

McCormick, E. Patricia, 494-95
McDermott, John F., 77, 103
Mace, David, 172
McLouth, Gary, 465
Madore, Carol, 382
Maes, John L., 435
Maguire, Daniel C., 99, 173
Maguire, Marjorie J., 173
Mahoney, Elizabeth, 119
Maine, Deborah, 383
Major, Brenda, 436

Mall, David, 437
Mallory, George B., 174
Mandel, Mark D., 100
Marder, Leon L., 438
Margolis, Alan J.,   101, 208, 247,
    323, 439
Marmer, Stephen S., 324
Martin, J.N., 272
Martindale, Lois J., 181
Mascovich, Paul R., 102
Mattingly, Richard F., 273
Maxton-Graham, Katrina, 440
Meyerowitz, Sanford, 441
Millard, Richard J., 157, 312
Miller, Eva, 274, 442
Miller, Warren B., 443
Moghadam, S.S., 275
Monsour, Karem J., 444
Moody, Howard, 306
Moore-Cavar, Emily C., 41
Morgentaler, Henry, 42
Morgenthau, Joan E., 179
Moseley, D.T., 445
Muhr, Janice Ruth, 175
Murphy, Maureen, 278

Nathanson, Bernard, 276-77
Nathanson, Constance A., 104-6
National Abortion Federation,
    43, 107
Naugle, Ethel, 325
Nazer, Isam R., 44
Ness, Mary, 326
Neubardt, Selig, 209
Newman, Lucille, 278
Nicholas, Nick, 408
Niswander, Kenneth, 446
Novak, F., 279

Olson, Lucy, 496
O'Neill, Patrick, 398
Oppel, Warren, 447
Ory, Warren, 447
Osofsky, Howard J., 45, 449
Osofsky, Joy D., 45, 449
Overstreet, E.W., 101

Pakter, Jean, 353
Paranjpe, M.K., 122
Pare, C.M.B., 450
Pasnau, Robert O., 451
Payne, E.D., 452
Pearson, J.F., 177
Penfield, A.J., 79, 280
Perez-Reyes, M., 453
Petchesky, Rosalind P., 46
Peterson, Herbert B., 353
Petres, Robert E., 3
Pike, M.C., 354
Pion, R.J., 110, 211
Piotrow, P.T., 291-93
Pipes, Mary, 47
Planned Parenthood Federation of
    America, 327
Planned Parenthood of New York
    City, Inc., 48
Poliak, Jose, 179
Potter, Robert G., 454
Potts, Malcolm, 50, 262
Pratt, Gail L., 111
Pritchard, Jack A., 51

Raven, H., 450
Reichelt, Paul A., 328
Resnik, H.L.P., 455
Richardson, John A., 385
Rifkin, John Robert, 456
Risk, Abraham, 213

Robbins, J.H., 457
Robbins, James M., 458-59
Roberts, G., 281
Robins, Sharon, 180
Robinson, Sharon E., 331
Roemer, Ruth, 113
Roht, Lewis H., 355, 386
Rooks, Judith Bourne, 282
Rosen, R.A., 114
Rosen, Raye Hudson, 181
Roth, Susan, 406
Rothstein, Arden A., 460
Rouse, B., 412
Rudel, Harry W., 52
Ryan, Ione J., 182

Sachs, Benjamin P., 356
Saltenberger, Ann, 214
Saltman, Jules, 53
Sanders, Raymond S., 329
Schiffer, M.A., 357
Schilling, Lee H., 461
Schneider, Sandra M., 183
Schoenbaum, S.C., 387
Schoenbucher, A.K., 360
Schonberg, Leonard A., 115
Schrader, Elinor S., 116
Schulder, Diane, 54
Schulman, Harold, 209, 283, 296
Schulz, Kenneth F., 146
Sciarra, John J., 55-56
Scott, Michael J., 57
Scotti, Richard J., 284
Seims, Sarah, 117
Selik, Richard M., 358
Selstad, Georgiana M., 462
Senay, Edward C., 463
Seward, Paul N., 359
Shalaby, Lynn M., 464

Shapiro, Howard I., 58
Shaw, Paul C., 184
Shelton, James D., 118, 360, 497
Shepard, Mary Jo, 185
Shostak, Arthur B., 465
Shusterman, Lisa R., 466, 498
Siegel, Mark, 59
Siener, Catherine H., 119
Sklar, June, 499
Skowronski, Marjory, 60
Slater, Paul E., 388
Sloane, R. Bruce, 61-62
Slome, John, 285
Smetana, Judith G., 186
Smith, E. Dorsey, 63
Smith, Elizabeth M., 330, 467
Smith, Mark Randall, 468
Smith, Roy, 80
Solberg, Norman, 246
Sood, S.V., 286
Southern, E.M., 253, 287
Speckhard, Annie Catherine, 469
Stallworthy, J.A., 23
Steege, J.F., 220
Steinhoff, Patricia G., 187
Steward, Barbara, 444
Stewart, Gary F., 361-2
Stim, Edward M., 288
Stroh, George, 289
Stubblefield, Phillip G., 290
Such-Baer, M., 121
Swartz, D.P., 122
Swigar, Mary E., 143

Tanner, Leonide M., 123
Theobald, Ellen M., 470
Thompson, Linda V., 331
Tietze, Christopher, 64-65
    188-90, 216, 227, 344, 471

Tinkham, Caroline B., 301
Todd, N.A., 472
Trichopoulos, D., 389

U.S. Department of Health, Education and Welfare. Center for Disease Control, 363
Ullmann, Alice, 332

Van den Vlugt, Theresa, 291-93
Vincent, L., 163

Waite, Ronald S., 259
Walbert, David F., 8
Wallerstein, Judith S., 473
Walter, George S., 474
Walton, Leslie A., 125
Watts, Walter F., 437
Weinstock, Edward, 126
Weisheit, Eldon, 191
Weiss, Theodore, 97
Wentz, Anne, 217
Werley, Harriet H., 328
West, N.D., 475
Westoff, Charles F., 476
Wheeler, R.G., 295
Whittington, H., 477
WHO Task Force on the Sequelae of Abortion, 390
WHO Task Force on the Use of Prostaglandins for the Regulation of Fertility, 294
Wickwire, Karen S., 333
Williams, Jean Morton, 478
Williford, J.F., 295
Wilson, Robert R., 334
Wittlin, Byron J., 455
Wolf, Sanford R., 127

Wolff, John R., 128
Women's Research Action Project, 129
Wong, Ting-Chao, 296
Wright, Charles S., 391
Wulff, George J.L. Jr., 130

Yaloff, Beverly, 131
Young, Alma T., 335
Young, Philip E., 132

Zatuchni, Gerald I., 66
Zellman, Gail L., 150
Zimering, Stanley, 53
Zimmerman, Mary K., 500

Title Index

Abortion, 50

Abortion (First Trimester), 218

Abortion: A Guide to Making Ethical Choices, 173

"Abortion: a social-psychological perspective," 395

"Abortion: a technique for working through grief," 304

Abortion: A Woman's Guide, 48

"Abortion, adoption or motherhood: an empirical study of
  decision-making during pregnancy," 13

Abortion: An Eternal Social and Moral Issue, 59

"Abortion: an issue to grieve?", 317

Abortion and Alternatives, 60

Abortion and Contraception, 42

Abortion and Contraception: A Study of Patient's Attitudes, 478

"Abortion and menstrual extraction for the ambulatory patient," 132

Abortion and Sterilization: Medical and Social Aspects, 32

Abortion and the Decision Not to Contracept, 170

Abortion and the Private Practice of Medicine, 92

"Abortion and psychological trauma," 425

"Abortion and sexual behavior in college women," 444

"Abortion and suicidal behaviors: observations on the concept of
  endangering the health of the mother," 455

Abortion and Woman's Choice: The State, Sexuality, and Reproductive
  Freedom, 46

"Abortion as 'deviance'--traditional female roles vs. the feminist
  perspective," 181

"Abortion as a treatment for unwanted pregnancy: the number two

sexually transmitted condition," 10
"Abortion attitudes among nurses and social workers," 89
"Abortion availability in the U.S.," 117
The Abortion Business: a Report on Free-Standing Abortion Clinics, 129
Abortion: Changing Views and Practice, 61
Abortion Clinic, 68
"The abortion constellation: early history and present relationships," 392
"Abortion counseling,"(Kahn-Edrington), 318
"Abortion counseling," (Brashaer), 303
"Abortion counseling,"(Asher), 299
"Abortion counseling: an experimental study of three techniques," 302
"Abortion counseling and behavioral change," 309
Abortion Counseling and Social Change, 306
"Abortion counseling: before, after, and again," 300
"Abortion counseling with adolescents," 311
"Abortion deaths associated with the use of PGFalpha," 336
"Abortion: do attitudes of nursing personnel affect the patient's perception of care?", 86
The Abortion Experience, 193
The Abortion Experience: Psychological and Medical Impact, 45
"Abortion facilities and the risk of death," 347
The Abortion Guide: A Handbook for Women and Men, 18
Abortion Handbook: History, Clinical Practice and Psychology of Abortion, 33
Abortion: Health Care Perspectives, 63
"Abortion, illegitimacy and the American birth rate," 499
"Abortion in psychological perspective," 409
Abortion in Psychosocial Perspective: Trends in Transnational Research, 483
Abortion in the Clinic and Office Setting, 87
Abortion in the Seventies, 30
"Abortion: Influences on health and professionals' attitudes," 73
"Abortion, is it a therapeutic procedure in psychiatry?", 414
Abortion: Law, Choice, and Morality, 9
"Abortion: liberal laws do make abortion safer for women," 15
Abortion: Listen to the Woman, 133
"Abortion: medical aspects in a municipal hospital," 122
Abortion: Medical Progress and Social Implication, 13
Abortion, Medicine and the Law, 8
"Abortion myths and realities: who is misleading whom?", 337

"Abortion needs and services in the United States," 126
"Abortion: physician and hospital attitudes," 85
Abortion Policy: an Evaluation of the Consequences for Maternal and Infant Health, 39
Abortion   Practice, 29
"Abortion: practice and promise," 207
Abortion Practice in Britain and the U.S., 21
"Abortion: predicting the complexity of the decision-making process," 155
"Abortion, psychiatry and the quality of life," 431
"Abortion: public health concerns and needed psychosocial research,"   484
Abortion Rap, 54
"Abortion repeal in Hawaii: an unexpected crisis in patient care," 103
"Abortion services in the United States, 1979 and 1980," 28
"Abortion: subjective attitudes and feelings," 153
Abortion Techniques and Services, 40
Abortion: The Agonizing Decision, 172
Abortion: The Emotional Implications, 426
Abortion: The Facts, 57
Abortion: The Personal Dilemma, 23
Abortion Today, 53
"Abortion under paracervical block," 280
"Abortion utilization: does travel distance matter?", 118
"Abortion without surgery?   Using prostaglandin F2alpha," 219
"Abortions and acute identity crisis in nurses," 77
"Abortions preventable by contraceptive practice," 476
"Additional births averted when abortion is added to contraception," 454
"Administrative guidelines for abortion service," 80
"Adolescent aborters: factors associated with gestational age," 179
"Adolescent abortions in the United States," 482
"Adolescent males, fatherhood, and abortion," 460
Adolescent Sexuality in a Changing American Society: Social and Psychological Perspectives, 12
"Advances in non-electrical vacuum equipment for uterine aspiration," 295
"Advice in the abortion decision," 171
After Abortion, 422
The Ambivalence of Abortion, 417
"Ambulatory abortion, experience with 26,000 cases," 276
"Anxiety-adjustment and other personality factors in teenage patients before and after abortion," 429

"An appraisal of abortion counseling," 326
"Areas of potential psychological vulnerability in the new era of liberalized abortion," 417
"Assessment of an intervention program for partners of abortion patients," 322
"Association of induced abortion with subsequent pregnancy loss," 378
"Assumption of attitudes toward abortion during physician education, 127
"Attributions, expectations, and coping with abortion," 436
"Attitudes of obstetric and gynecologic residents toward abortion," 102
"Attitudes of women who have had abortions," 403
Attitudes toward Abortion, 494

"Behavioral factors contributing to abortion deaths: a new approach to mortality studies," 358
Birth Control and Abortion, 471
The Birth Control Book, 58
Birth Control, Contraception and Abortion, 52
"Birth control use by teenagers: one and two years postabortion," 393
"Brief communication: psychological reactions to abortion," 405

A Case Study of the Reproductive Experience of Women Who Have Had Three or More Induced Abortions, 169
"Characteristics of women recruited to a long-term study of the sequelae of induced abortion," 492
"Clinical experience in using intraamniotic PGF2alpha for midtrimester abortion in 600 patients," 220
Clinical Use of Prostaglandins for Pregnancy Termination, 234
"College students' attitudes toward shared responsibility in decisions about abortion: implications for counseling," 182
"The comparative efficacy and safety of intraamniotic prostaglandin F2alpha and hypertonic saline for second trimester abortion," 252
"Comparative risk of death from induced abortion at less than 12 weeks' gestation," 353
"Comparative risks of three methods of mid-trimester abortion," 363
"A comparative study of recidivists and contraceptors along the dimensions of locus of control and impulsivity," 156
"Comparison of intraamniotic prostaglandin F2alpha and hypertonic saline

for induction of second-trimester abortion," 294
"A comparison of metal and plastic cannulae for performing vacuum aspiration during the first trimester of pregnancy," 275
Comparison of the Medical Effects of Induced Abortion by Two Methods: Curettage and Vacuum Aspiration, 279
"Comparison of women seeking early and late abortion," 151
"Competing risks of unnecessary procedures and complications," 245
"Complications of outpatient abortion," 115
"Components of delay amongst women obtaining termination of pregnancy," 135
"Concept of quality care in abortion services," 90
A Consumer's Guide to Deception, Harassment and Medical Malpractice, 327
"Contraception, abortion, and VD," 328
Contraception, Abortion, Pregnancy, 205
"Contraception after abortion," 439
"Contraception immediately post-abortion," 421
"Contraceptive antecedents to early and late therapeutic abortions," 447
"Contraceptive practice and repeat induced abortion," 185
"Connecticut physicians' attitudes toward abortion," 111
Concepts of Self and Morality: Women's Reasoning About Abortion, 186
"The consequences of abortion legislation," 7
"Consequences of induced abortion," 368
"Coordination of outpatient services for patients seeking elective abortion," 119
"Coping with abortion," 406
"Counseling abortion patients," 325
"Counseling for elective abortion," 329
"Counseling for women who seek abortion," 330
Counseling in Abortion Services: Physician-Nurse-Social Worker, 307
"Counseling the abortion patient is more than talk," 319
"Counseling women who are considering abortion," 320
"Counselling needs of women seeking abortions," 315
"Counselling of patients requesting abortion," 310
"Creating and controlling a medical market," 84
"Current status of the use of prostaglandins in induced abortion," 240

" D & E midtrimester abortion: a medical innovation," 269
"Deaths after legally induced abortion," 360

"Deaths from second trimester abortion by dilatation and evacuation," 338
"The decision-making process and the outcome of therapeutic abortion,"
    419
"The decision to abort and psychological sequelae," 140
"Delayed abortion in an area of easy accessability," 146
A Descriptive Study of the Attitudes of Males Involved in Abortion, 147
The Determinants of Psychological Response to Abortion, 411
"Developing professional parameters," 123
"Development of an abortion service in a large municipal hospital," 125
"Differences in self-concept and locus of control among women who
    seek abortions," 331
A Difficult Decision: A Compassionate Book about Abortion, 22
"Dilatation and curettage for second-trimester abortions," 256
"Dilatation and evacuation: a preferred method of midtrimester abortion,"
    235
"Dilatation and evacuation at 13 to 15 weeks' gestation versus intra-
    amniotic saline after 15 weeks' gestation," 230
"Dilatation and evacuation procedures and second-trimester abortions:the
    role of physician skill and hospital setting," 236
"Divergent perspectives in abortion counseling," 312
A Doctor's Guide to Having an Abortion, 26
"Does abortion affect later pregnancies?", 383
"Drugs for the production of abortion: a review," 277

"Early abortion in a family planning clinic," 83
Early Abortion: The Earlier the Better, 242
"Early complications and late sequelae of induced abortion," 345
"Early second trimester abortion by the extraamniotic instillation of
    Rivanol solution and a single PGF2alpha dose," 272
"Early vacuum aspiration: minimizing procedures to nonpregnant women,"
    274
Eclipse of Reason, 203
"Ectopic pregnancy and prior induced abortion," 379
"The effect of delay and choice of method on the risk of abortion
    morbidity," 339
Effect of Induced Abortion on Subsequent Reproductive Function, 381
"Effect of legal abortion on the rate of septic abortion at a large county
    hospital," 359
"Effect of legalized abortion on morbidity resulting from criminal

abortion," 349

"Effect of liberalized abortion on maternal mortality rates," 340

"The effect of method of abortion on the outcome of subsequent pregnancies," 388

"The effectiveness and complications of abortion by dilatation and vacuum aspiration versus dilatation and rigid metal curettage," 243

"The effects of induced abortion on subsequent reproduction," 373

Effects of Induced Abortion on Subsequent Reproductive Functions and Pregnancy Outcome, 366

"Effects of legal termination on subsequent pregnancy," 385

"Efficacy of a group crisis-counseling program for men who accompany women seeking abortions," 314

"Efficiency of menstrual regulation as a method of fertility control," 227

"Elective abortion: complications seen in a freestanding clinic," 130

"Emotional distress patterns among women having first or repeat abortions," 154

"Emotional impact of D & E versus instillation," 282

"Emotional patterns related to delay in decision to seek legal abortion," 165

"Emotional reactions in abortion service personnel," 94

"Emotional responses of women following therapeutic abortion," 396

"Endometrial aspiration as a means of early abortion," 296

"Endometrial aspiration in fertility control," 223

An Epidemiological Study of Psychosocial Correlates of Delayed Decisions to Abort, 141

"Equity in abortion services," 113

"Evaluating the quality of abortion services by measuring outcomes," 76

"Evaluation of abortion techniques," 211

"Evaluation of abortion: techniques and protocols," 198

"Evaluation of therapeutic abortion as an element of preventative psychiatry," 477

Everything you Need to Know About Abortion, 27

Every Woman Has a Right to Know the Dangers of Legal Abortion, 214

Every-Woman's Guide to Abortion, 19

Experience with Abortion, 490

Fact Sheet Series, 43

"Factors affecting gestational age at termination of pregnancy," 163

"Factors associated with delay in seeking induced abortion," 142

"Factors predicting pregnancy resolution decision satisfaction of unmarried adolescents," 150

"Factors related to delay for legal abortions performed at a gestational age of 20 weeks or more," 164

"Factors responsible for delay in obtaining interruption of pregnancy," 174

"Factors to consider in staffing an abortion service facility," 70

Fertility Control, 201

"First and repeat abortions: a study of decision-making and delay," 143

"First-trimester induced abortion," 208

"Five thousand consecutive saline inductions," 264

Five Young Women, 152

"Follow-up after therapeutic abortion in early adolescence," 453

"Follow-up of patients recommended for therapeutic abortion," 472

"A follow-up study of women who request abortion," 467

"Free standing abortion clinics: a new phenomenon," 88

A General Guide to Abortion, 62

"Gestation, birthweight, and spontaneous abortion in pregnancy after induced abortion," 390

"Group therapy following abortion," 301

Gynecology and Obstetrics, 55

Having a Wonderful Abortion, 180

"Health professionals' attitudes toward abortion," 114

"Health professionals' perceptions of the psychological consequences of abortion," 398

"Hospitalization for medical-legal and other abortions in the U.S.:1970-1977," 6

How Men who Accompany Women to an Abortion Service Perceive the Impact of Abortion Upon their Relationships and Themselves, 468

How Women Feel About Abortion: Psychological, Attitudinal and Physical Effects of Legal Abortion, 464

"Human rights in relationship to induced abortion," 188

"Husbands of abortion applicants: a comparison with husbands of women who complete their pregnancies," 434

"Impact of legal abortion: redefining the maternal mortality rate," 355

"Impact of the abortion experience on contraceptive acceptance," 442

"Impact of the liberalized abortion law in New York City on deaths associated with pregnancy," 353

"Impact of vacuum aspiration abortion on future childbearing," 374

In Necessity and Sorrow: Life and Death in an Abortion Hospital, 16

Induced Abortion (Kleinman), 37

"Induced abortion" (Tietze), 64

Induced Abortion: a Hazard to Public Health?, 44

Induced Abortion: A World Review, 65

"Induced abortion after feeling fetal movements," 144

"Induced abortion and its sequelae," 386

"Induced abortion and secondary infertility," 389

"Induced abortion and spontaneous abortion: no connection?", 377

"Induced abortion and spontaneous fetal loss in subsequent pregancies," 367

"Induced abortion and sterilization among women who became mothers as adolescents," 162

"Induced abortion and subsequent outcome of pregnancy in a series of American women," 371

"Induced abortion as a risk factor for perinatal complications," 363

"Induced abortion for psychiatric indications," 441

Induced Abortion: Guidelines for the Provision of Care and Services, 93

"Induced abortion: source of guilt or growth?", 297

"The induction of mid-trimester abortion with intra-amniotic prostaglandin F2alpha: a single dose technique," 239

"Induction of midtrimester abortion with intraamniotic urea, intravenous oxytocin and laminaria," 246

"Induction of therapeutic abortion by intra-amniotic injection of urea," 248

"Influence of induced and spontaneous abortion on the outcome of subsequent pregnancies," 384

"Influence of personality attributes on abortion experiences," 418

"The interactive effects of induced abortion, inter-pregnancy interval and contraceptive use on subsequent pregnancy outcome," 375

International Inventory of Information on Induced Abortion, 41

Interruption of Pregnancy--A Total Patient Approach, 4

"An investigation of the abortion decision process," 184

"Is psychiatric consultation in abortion obsolete?", 324

It Happens to Us, 35

"JPSA for the study of abortion: early medical complications of legal abortion," 216

"The Karman catheter: a preliminary evaluation," 226
"King's termination study II" 399

"Late effects of induced abortion," 365
"Late sequelae of induced abortion," 372
"Learning abortion care," 82
"Legal abortion reduces out-of-wedlock births," 493
"Legal abortion: the public health record," 11
"Legal abortion without hospitalization," 101
"Legal abortions and trends in age-specific marriage rates," 480
Legalized Abortion and the Public Health, 34
"Legalized abortion: effect on national trends of maternal and abortion-related mortality rates," 341
"Low birthweight subsequent to induced abortion," 376

"Major complications of 20,248 consecutive first trimester abortions," 348
Making Choices: Evaluating the Health Risks and Benefits of Birth Control Methods, 448
"Management of midtrimester abortion failures by vaginal evacuation," 232
"Mass-produced assembly-line abortion," 416
A Matter of Choice: An Essential Guide to Every Aspect of Abortion, 17
"Medical and surgical complications of therapeutic abortions," 361
Men and Abortion: Losses, Lessons, and Love, 465
Men and the Abortion Experience, 432
"Menstrual extraction" (Atienza), 221
"Menstrual extraction" (Hodgson), 257
"Menstrual induction," 247
"Menstrual induction: its place in clinical practice," 260
"Menstrual induction: II. Psycho-social aspects," 278
"Menstrual regulation and early pregnancy termination," 284
"Menstrual regulation in family planning service," 265
"Menstrual regulation in the U.S.," 229

"Menstrual regulation update," 291
"Menstrual regulation/vacuum abortion: a valid distinction?", 238
"Menstrual regulation: what is it?", 292
'Midtrimester abortion," 206
"Mid-trimester abortion" (Finks), 244
"Mid-trimester abortion" (Davis), 241
"Midtrimester abortion by D & E," 249
"Midtrimester abortion by D & E versus intra-amniotic instillation of prostaglanding F2alpha," 250
"Midtrimester abortion by intraamniotic prostaglandin F2alpha," 251
"Midtrimester abortion induced with a single intra-amniotic instillation of prostaglandin F2alpha," 266
"Mid-trimester abortion: 12 to 20 weeks by dilatation and evacuation method," 222
"Monitoring care in abortion clinics," 96
More than a Choice,20
"Mortality associated with hypertonic saline abortion," 357
"Mortality from abortion and childbirth," 350
"Mortality from abortion and childbirth: are the populations comparable?," 351
"Mortality from abortion and childbirth: are the statistics biased?", 342

"A naturalistic study of abortion decisions," 158
New Concepts in Contraception, 75
The New Our Bodies, Ourselves, 5
New Perspectives in Human Abortion, 31
A New View of a Woman's Body, 204
"Nurses' feelings a problem under new abortion law," 108
"Nursing care in an abortion unit," 131

"OB/GYN nurse group takes stand on abortion," 109
"OR nurses face decision in abortion procedures," 116
"Objective vs. subjective responses to abortion," 457
"Obstetricians' attitudes and hospital abortion services," 104
"An operational and planning staffing model for first and second trimester abortion services," 100
"Oral contraceptive use and early abortion as risk factors for breast cancer in young women," 354

"Organizing an abortion service," 78
"Outcome following therapeutic abortion," 452
"Outcome of the delivery following an induced or spontaneous abortion," 387
"Out-of-wedlock abortion and delivery," 450
"Outpatient saline abortion," 283
"Outpatient second-trimester D & E abortion," 255
"Outpatient termination of pregnancy," 268
"Outsiders' reactions to abortion," 81
"Oxytocin administration, instillation-to-abortion time, and morbidity associated with saline instillation," 224

"The paramedic abortionist" (Mattingly), 273
"The paramedic abortionist" (Karman), 95
"Patterns of discussion and decision-making amongst abortion patients," 136
Personal Decisions, 178
Personality Correlates of the Delayed Abortion Decision, 148
"Personality factors related to black teenage pregnancy and abortion," 486
Personality Factors, Self-Concept, and Family Variables related to First-Time and Repeat Abortion-Seeking Behavior in Adolescent Women, 485
"Physician behavior as a determinant of utilization patterns," 105
"Physicians' attitudes toward abortion," 98
Physiology of Miscarriage and Abortion, 210
"Pilot study of single women requesting a legal abortion,"177
Planned Parenthood Response to 'The Silent Scream', 212
Point Counterpoint, 49
"A portrait of American women who obtain abortions," 489
"Post-abortion attitudes and patterns of birth control," 394
"Post-abortion group therapy," 305
A Post-Abortion Study and Attitude Comparison of Women who had and had not given Birth to Living Children, 470
"Postcoital contraception," 461
"Postpartum and postabortion psychotic reactions," 410
Pre-Abortion Psychological Experience and its Relationship to Post-Abortion Psychological Outcome, 424
"Predicting contraceptive use in postabortion patients," 462

"Predicting the psychological consequences of abortion," 466
"Predictive factors in emotional response to abortion," 400
Pregnancy, Birth, and Family Planning, 24
"Pregnancy termination in midtrimester," 200
Pregnancy Termination: Procedures, Safety and New Developments, 66
"Preventing unwanted pregnancies," 110
Pregnant by Mistake: The Stories of Seventeen Women, 440
"The 'problem' of repeat abortions," 189
Problem Pregnancy and Abortion Counseling, 334
"Professional norms, personal attitudes and medical practice," 106
"Professional staff reaction to abortion work," 121
"Psychiatric complications of therapeutic abortion," 451
"Psychiatric experience with a liberalized abortion law," 438
"Psychiatric sequelae of legalized elective first trimester abortion," 430
"Psychiatric sequelae to term birth and induced early and late abortion,"
   397
"Psychiatric sequelae to therapeutic abortion," 450
"Psychological and emotional consequences of elective abortion," 474
Psychological Adjustment to First Trimester Abortion, 175
"Psychological and social aspects of induced abortion," 487
Psychological Aspects of Abortion, 437
"Psychological consequences of adolescent pregnancy and abortion," 433
"Psychological factors in mid-trimester abortion," 166
"Psychological factors involved in request for elective abortion," 138
"Psychological factors that predict reaction to abortion," 445
"Psychological impact of abortion," 475
"Psychological reaction of patients to legalized abortion," 449
"Psychological reaction to therapeutic abortion," 446
"Psychological sequelae of abortion," 413
"Psychological sequelae of abortion performed for genetic indication,"
   402
"Psychological vulnerability to unwanted pregnancy," 443
"Psychosocial aspects of abortion," 491
"Psychosocial aspects of fertility regulation," 495
"Psychosocial consequences of therapeutic abortion," 423
"Psychosocial factors of the abortion experience," 498
"Psychosocial sequelae of therapeutic abortion in young unmarried
   women," 473

"The RN panel of 500 tells what nurses think about abortion," 112

"Randomized study of 12mm and 15.9 canullas in midtrimester abortion," 290

"Reasons for delayed abortion," 167

"Reassessment of menstrual regulation," 258

"Recommended program guide for abortion services," 72

Reflections of a Catholic Theologian on Visiting an Abortion Clinic, 99

"The relationship between induced abortion and outcome of subsequent pregnancies," 380

"Relationship between legal abortion and marriage," 481

"Relationships among knowledge, attitudes and behavior of nurses concerning abortion," 69

Relationships and Abortion, 456

"Repeat aborters," 183

"The repeat abortion patient," 168

"Repeat abortion--why more?", 190

"Repeat abortions: blaming the victims," 160

Report of the Committee on the Working of the Abortion Act, 38

"Reported live births following induced abortion," 289

"Reproductive mortality in the U.S.," 356

"Research on repeated abortion," 157

"Response to requests for abortion," 134

"Results in 1000 cases of therapeutic abortion managed by vacuum aspiration," 271

"A review of one thousand uncomplicated vaginal operations for abortion," 196

The Right to Abortion: A Psychiatric View, 159

Risks, Benefits, and Controversies in Fertility Control, 56

"Role of induced abortion in secondary infertility," 369

"The role of private counseling for problem pregnancies," 298

"The role of the nurse-midwife in an abortion evaluation clinic," 67

The Safety of Fertility Control, 36

"Saline abortion," 288

Second Trimester Abortion, 195

"Second trimester abortion after vaginal termination of pregnancy," 391

"Second trimester abortion in the United States," 194

"Second trimester abortions: review of four procedures," 213

"Second trimester interruption of pregnancy," 197

Second Trimester Pregnancy Termination, 263
"Selected psychosocial characteristics of males," 479
"Self-administration of prostaglandin for termination of early pregnancy," 233
"Sex guilt in abortion patients," 420
"Sexuality, birth control and abortion: a decision-making sequence," 149
"Short-term psychiatric sequelae to therapeutic termination of pregnancy," 428
"Should family planning clinics perform abortions?", 79
"Should I have an abortion?", 191
Silent Scream, 215
"Social and psychological correlates of pregnancy resolution among adolescent women," 496
"Social work service to abortion patients," 332
"Some thoughts on medical evaluation and counseling of applicants for abortion," 323
"Standardized mortality rates associated with legal abortion," 344
Standards for Abortion Services, 107
Standards for Obstetric-Gynecologic Services, 71
"A statement on abortion by one hundred professors of obstetrics," 120
"Sterilization associated with induced abortion," 270
"A study of abortion and problems in decision-making," 308
"A study on the effects of induced abortion on subsequent pregnancy outcome," 382
Subsequent Pregnancy Outcome following Induced Abortion, 370
"Successful first trimester abortion following the use of 15(S) 15-methyl-prostaglandin F2alpha methyl ester vaginal suppositories," 228
"Sudden collapse and death of women obtaining abortions induced with prostaglandin F2alpha," 343
"A suggested set of working definitions and criteria applicable to interruption of pregnancy," 1
"Support from significant others and loneliness following induced abortion," 459

Techniques of Abortion, 209
"Techniques of induced abortion: their health implications and service aspects," 346
"Techniques of pregnancy termination," 217
"Techiques of pregnancy termination, part II," 199

"The termination of human pregnancy with prostaglandin analogs," 253
"Termination of pregnancy," 285
"Termination of pregnancy by 'super coils,'" 225
"Termination of pregnancy by the interuterine insertion of Utus paste,"
  286
"Termination of pregnancy in a private outpatient clinic," 74
"Therapeutic abortion and a prior psychiatric history," 412
"Therapeutic abortion: attitudes of medical personnel leading to
  complications in patient care," 128
"Therapeutic abortion by intra-amniotic injection of prostaglandins," 281
"Therapeutic abortion: clinical aspects," 463
"Therapeutic abortion in California," 362
"Therapeutic abortion using prostagladin F2," 261
"Therapeutic abortion: who needs a psychiatrist," 415
Thinking About Abortion, 401
"Third time unlucky: a study of women who have had three or more legal
  abortions," 145
"33,000 doctors speak out on abortion," 124

Understanding Abortion, 47
"Unmarried Black adolescent fathers' attitudes toward abortion,
  contraception, and sexuality," 488
Unwanted Pregnancies Terminated by Induced Abortion: A Study in
  Unconscious Motivational Factors, 404
The Unwanted Pregnancy, 3
The Use of Behavioral Intervention in the Preparation of Patients for the
  Surgical Procedure Involved in Pregnancy Termination, 333
"Use of conception control methods before pregnancies terminating in
  birth or a requested abortion in New York City municipal hospitals," 408
"The use of prostaglandins for the therapeutic termination of pregnancy,"
  287
"Uterine aspiration techniques," 293
Uterine Aspiration Techniques in Family Planning, 259

"Vacuum aspiration of the uterus in therapeutic abortion," 231
"Vaginal administration of prostaglandins to induce early abortion," 254
"Vaginal hysterectomy," 267
"Variables in abortion counseling," 313

"Very early abortion using syringe as vacuum source," 262

"Very young adolescent women in Georgia: has abortion or contraception lowered their fertility," 497

Voluntary Termination of Pregnancy, 25

"Ward staff problems with abortions," 97

"What abortion counselors want from their clients," 316

What Every Woman Needs to Know About Abortion, 2

Williams Obstetrics, 51

Woman's Body: An Owner's Manual, 202

A Woman's Choice, 137

A Woman's Guide to Safe Abortion, 14

Women Who Have Had an Abortion, 192

"Women who obtain repeat abortions," 187

"Women who seek abortions," 335

"Women's responses to abortion: implications for post-abortion support groups," 321

"World Health Organization studies of prostaglandins versus saline as abortifacients," 237

Subject Index

Abortifacients, 277. *See also* Specific names of abortifacients

Abortion (general), 1-66

Abortion, complications. *See* Morbidity and mortality

Abortion, early. *See* Abortion, first trimester

Abortion, elective. *See* name of specific area of interest

Abortion, first trimester: and birth control, 394, 399; complications of, 115, 130, 348; development of techniques, 207-8; dilatation and curettage (D & C), 68, 74, 243, 262, 274-75, 280; evaluation of techniques, 211, 217-18; and family planning clinics, 79;

menstrual regulation, 226, 228, 265, 284, 296; outpatient, 268; physicians and, 83; prostaglandins, 233-34, 240, 254; psychological factors, 175, 400, 406, 423, 436, 445; psychosocial factors, 167, 173; staffing model for, 100. *See also* Abortion techniques (general); Abortion techniques (specific)

Abortion, incidence of *See* Epidemiology

Abortion, late. *See* Abortion, second trimester

Abortion, midtrimester. *See* Abortion, second trimester

Abortion, second trimester, 194-95, 197; delay in obtaining, 163-64, 167, 174;

dilatation and curettage (D & C),256; dilatation and suction evacuation (D & E), 203, 222 235-36, 241, 250-51, 255; equipment, 290; failures, 232; mortality, 338, 357; prostaglandins, 219-20, 234, 239-40, 248, 252, 266; risks, 363; staffing model, 100; techniques, 36, 199-200, 206-7, 211, 213, 244, 246, 263, 272, 294. *See also* Abortion techniques (general); Abortion techniques (specific)

Abortion, therapeutic. *See* name of specific area of interest

Abortion accessability, 3, 113, 117-18, 126

Abortion availability, 3, 113, 117-18, 126

Abortion clinics, 67-132; description, 5; evaluation, 14, 16, 192, 327; list of, 18; mortality rates, 347

Abortion deaths. *See* Morbidity and mortality

Abortion decision, 133-91, 478

Abortion effects on subsequent pregnancy, 25, 36, 363-90

Abortion facilities. *See* Abortion clinics

Abortion techniques(general), 2-5, 13, 17-18, 24-26, 29, 31-32, 35, 41-42, 45, 47-48, 50-53, 56-58, 63-64, 66, 87, 93, 193-217, 334

Abortion techniques (specific), 74, 101, 115, 218-96

Adolescents (and abortion), 12; contraception, 328, 393, 497; counseling, 311, 453; delay in obtaining abortions, 179; epidemiology, 482; male partners and, 460, 488; pregnancy, 49; psychological aspects, 429; psychosocial factors, 485-86, 496

Alternatives (to abortion), 2, 17, 20, 22, 60, 139, 334

Ambulatory clinics: abortion, first trimester, 101; complications, 130; description, 88, 119, 125, 129; saline abortion, 283; standards, 71, 132; statistical data, 276. *See also* Abortion clinics

Anesthesia. *See* Abortion techniques (general) ; Abortion techniques (specific)

Anti-abortion viewpoint, 31, 57, 68, 203, 214-5, 416, 437

Behavioral intervention, 333

Birth control. *See* Contraception
Birthweight, 375, 382, 387, 389.
See also Abortion effects on
subsequent pregnancy

Breast cancer (and abortion), 11

Cancer, breast (and abortion), 11

College students (and abortion),
182, 329, 444

Complications. *See* Abortion
techniques (general); Abortion
techniques (specific); Morbidity
and Mortality

Contraception: and adolescents,
393, 497; breast cancer, risk
of, 354; choice, 75; counseling,
137, 298, 319, 320, 334;
epidemiology, 34; failure, 49,
138, 145; fertility regulation,
201; international aspects, 42;
male partners and, 322, 479;
post-abortion, 2, 63, 242, 263,
399, 421, 439; post-coital
(PCC), 58; and pregnancy,
subsequent, 375, 453;
psychosocial aspects, 495; and
risk-taking, 170; risks of, 448;
sexuality, 149; sterilization, 32;
techniques, 14, 17-18, 20, 27,
43, 48, 52, 55, 60, 205, 471;
usage, 185, 408, 442, 447, 462,

476, 478

Contraceptive choice [before and
after abortion]. *See*
Contraception

Contraceptive use [before and
after abortion]. *See*
Contraception

Costs (of abortion). *See*
Economics of abortion

Counseling, 4, 30, 66, 87, 137,
172, 297-335; and college
students, 181; guidelines, 93;
outpatient clinics, 75, 79. *See
also* Psychological effects

Counselor, attitudes, 215

Curettage *See* Dilatation and
curettage

Deaths, abortion. *See* Morbidity
and mortality

Delay in obtaining abortions,
263, 339

Demographic aspects (of
abortion), 4, 5, 8, 11, 34, 40,
55, 65, 263

Denied abortion, 24, 409

Dilatation and curettage (D & C),
74, 215, 243, 256, 364, 388.

See also Abortion techniques (specific)

Dilatation and suction evacuation (D & E): abortion, first trimester, 280; abortion, second trimester, 250-51, 269; anti-abortion viewpoint, 215; complications, 230, 235, 243, 348; outpatient, 255; psychological effects, 282, techniques, 222, 285. *See also* Abortion techniques (specific)

Economics, 20, 43, 53

Ectopic pregnancy, 378

Endometrial aspiration. *See* Menstrual regulation

Epidemiology: contraceptive practice, 185; incidence of abortion, 25, 28-30, 59, 64-65, 216; males, 479; marriage rates, 480; pregnancy, subsequent, 366-67, 370-1, 380-1; techniques, 238

Ethical considerations, 27, 40, 176

Evaluation of abortion services, 29-30, 76, 90, 122, 198

Family, abortion effects on, 53, 459

Family planning, 37, 83, 110.*See also* Contraception; Psychological effects

Fathers (and abortion): adolescents, 460, 488; attitudes, college students,182; counseling, 314, 322; decision-making, 147, 184; psychological effects, 432, 459; and relationships, 456, 458, 468; psychosocial aspects, 433, 479

Fertility choice. *See* Contraception; psychological effects

Fetal development, 17, 49, 57

Gestalt technique, 303

Great Britain, abortion in, 21, 38, 50, 57

Group therapy, 301, 304, 314, 321, 332

Health professionals. *See* Staffing

Hospitals and abortion, 85, 103, 236, 347, 484. *See also* Abortion clinics

Intraamniotic techniques. *See* name of specific technique or abortifacient

Laminaria tents, 246, 255, 285, 290

Law, abortion, 8-9, 11, 21, 26, 30, 33, 42, 44, 64, 87; and criminal abortion, 349; history of, 62-64, 320; and public health, 11, 34, 352; safety, 15, 31, 337, 340-1, 344, 354

Legislation, abortion, 7, 30, 37, 64 Live births (following induced abortion), 13, 237, 289

Male partners (and abortion). *See* Fathers (and abortion)

Marriage, effects of abortion on, 13

Menstrual extraction. *See* Menstrual regulation

Menstrual induction. *See* Menstrual regulation

Menstrual regulation: ambulatory abortion, 132; definition, 257; evaluation, 223, 227, 229, 238, 247, 258, 260, 291-2; and

family planning, 83, 265 ; psychosocial aspects, 278; risks, 245; techniques, 36, 56, 211, 221, 284, 296. *See also* Abortion techniques (general); Abortion techniques (specific)

Middle East, abortion in, 44

Mini-suction. *See* Abortion techniques (specific)

Morbidity and Mortality, 25, 32, 36, 42-43, 286, 336-63; complications, 51, 63, 235, 251, 273, 293; epidemiology, 216; outpatient termination, 75, 115, 125, 196; public health, 34; saline abortion, 224, 264; second trimester, 194, 225, 256; statistics, 50, 64-65, 87 *See also* Abortion techniques (general); Abortion techniques (specific)

Mortality .*See* Morbidity and mortality

Nurses, attitudes, 69, 89, 112, 114, 121; professional guidelines, 109, 116; psychological reactions, 77, 94, 103, 108; quality of care, 86, 123; staffing, 70. *See* also Abortion clinics

Nursing (of abortion patients),

30, 67-70, 82, 86, 131. *See also* Abortion clinics

Outpatient abortion. *See* Ambulatory abortion

Oxytocin abortion, 224, 246, 268. *See also* Abortion techniques (specific).

PCC *See* Postcoital contraception

Paramedics, 95, 273, 283. *See also* Abortion clinics

Parents (of abortion patients), 178

Pastoral counseling .*See* Counseling

Patient screening, 29

Physicians, attitudes, 68, 84-85, 92, 102, 111, 397; education, 127; involvement in abortion issues, 120, 124, 431; psychological reactions, 94, 121; quality of care, 104-5, 128. *See also* Abortion clinics

Physicians, training and/or practice in abortion techniques, 92, 94, 127, 236, 238

Policy (abortion), 39

Political aspects of abortion, 29

Post-abortion complications *See* Abortion techniques (specific); Morbidity and mortality; Sequelae of abortion

Postcoital contraception, 58, 217, 460. *See also* Abortion techniques (specific)

Pregnancy, abortion effects on subsequent, 25, 36, 363-90

Pregnancy, illegitimate, 23, 177, 458, 472, 492, 499

Pregnancy, physiology, 63, 259

Pregnancy tests, 14, 66, 245, 257-58, 260, 274

Prostaglandin abortion: evaluation, 235, 237, 240, 253, 256, 294; first trimester abortion, 228, 254; morbidity and mortality, 335, 338, 342; second trimester abortion, 207, 213, 220, 239, 250-2, 266; self-administered, 233; techniques, 36, 56, 198, 219, 234, 261, 272, 281, 287. *See also* Abortion techniques (specific)

Psychiatric evaluation, 324, 414-15, 438, 441, 463

Psychiatric hospitalization, 13

Psychological effects, 2, 4-5, 12, 17-18, 22, 26, 30, 41-42, 45, 49, 57, 193, 392-478; adjustment, 47, 175; delayed abortion, 148; decision-making, 140, 142, 149; fetal movement, 144; mental health, 32, 154; public health aspects, 34; second trimester abortion, 166

Psychosocial aspects, 12, 25, 37, 44, 397, 403, 473, 479-500; decision-making, 139, 149, 435; delayed decision, 141, 143, 151, 174; genetic indications, 402; menstrual induction, 287; morbidity and mortality, 360; repeat aborters, 161, 185; socioeconomic trends, 45, 57, 62

Referral agencies. *See* Counseling

Refused abortion, consequences of, 23, 409

Religious considerations, 27, 41, 53, 173, 422

Repeat abortions, 409, 485. *See also* Abortion decision; Psychological effects

Saline abortion: evaluation, 213, 237, 251-2, 256, 288, 294; live births, 289; morbidity and

mortality, 357; outpatient, 283; risks, 207, 224, 230, 264. *See also* Abortion techniques (specific)

Scotland, abortion in, 489

Self-induced abortion, 233

Septic abortion. *See* Abortion techniques (general); Abortion techniques (specific); Morbidity and mortality

Septic shock. *See* Abortion techniques (general); Abortion techniques (specific); Morbidity and mortality

Sequelae of abortion, 13-14, 29, 50, 65, 140, 365, 492. *See also* Abortion techniques (general); Abortion techniques (specific); Pregnancy, abortion effects on subsequent; Psychological effects

Sex and sexuality , 20, 46, 55, 149, 420, 444, 478-79. *See also* Psychological effects

Sexual behavior, abortion influence on subsequent. *See* Psychological effects

Social workers, 89, 121, 123, 397. *See also* Counseling

Socioeconomic aspects. *See* Psychosocial aspects

Staffing (of abortion facility), 29, 70, 73, 91, 97, 114, 123

Staffing attitudes, 69, 72, 90, 96, 113, 122

Standards for abortion services, 72, 80, 93, 107, 259; ambulatory facilities, 71, 131; monitoring, 96; nurses, 109; staffing, 100

Sterilization and abortion, 4, 26, 55, 93, 270; adolescents, 162; techniques, 32, 267. *See also* Abortion techniques (specific)

Suction aspiration. *See* Vacuum aspiration

"Super coils," 225, 273

Terminology, 1, 40, 51-52

Therapeutic abortion. *See* name of specific area of interest

United Kingdom, abortion in, 21, 38, 50, 57

Unwanted pregnancy. *See* Abortion decision

Urea abortion, 246, 248, 255

Uterine aspiration. *See* Vacuum aspiration

Utus paste abortion, 286

Vacuum aspiration: equipment, 295; evaluation, 271; family planning, 259; morbidity and mortality, 363; paraprofessionals, 284; pregnancy, effects on, 374; second trimester, 230; techniques, 208, 218, 231-32, 238, 262, 274-75, 290, 293. *See also* Abortion techniques (specific)

Venereal disease, 10

About the Compiler

EUGENIA B. WINTER is Acquisitions Librarian/Bibliographer at California State College, Bakersfield.